# TREATING BODY, MIND AND SOUL

# BY THE SAME AUTHOR

*Healthcare* series

# TREATING BODY, MIND AND SOUL

## Jan de Vries

MAINSTREAM
PUBLISHING
EDINBURGH AND LONDON

First published in Great Britain in 2003 by
MAINSTREAM PUBLISHING (EDINBURGH) LTD
7 Albany Street
Edinburgh EH1 3UG

ISBN 1 84018 463 9

A catalogue record for this book is available from the British Library

Typeset in Bembo and Book Antiqua

Printed in Great Britain by
Creative Print & Design Wales

# CONTENTS

# BODY

Throughout the 45 years I have studied the body and its marvellous construction, I have been constantly amazed at how it works. It is so beautiful and harmonious, and it would take a whole library of books to thoroughly discuss every part. In the 40 that I have written, I have only given a glimpse of what the body really is. We can only observe in astonishment when thousands of agents come to help heal even a little cut. Sometimes just an incredibly small adjustment is all that is needed to improve one's health. I find it remarkable to see how the body heals itself if sensible steps are taken. On the other hand, it is also unbelievable how many people destroy their own bodies through neglect.

When I see patients, I remember what I was taught during my time in China – to look, to listen and to feel. I can generally make a diagnosis even before a patient sits down before me in the consulting room. By looking at the placement of the ears and observing any imbalances the patient may have developed, I can consider where things have gone wrong in the body and decide what to do to harmonise it. The body can be likened to a ship that is overburdened on one side and capsizes, or the smallest wheel in a watch that fails to turn properly and stops the watch from ticking. Even minor problems can disturb the balance of our body and hinder it from working efficiently.

Chinese facial diagnosis, which I learned many years ago, is one of the tools that allow me to pinpoint problems so quickly. Using facial diagnosis, I can *look* and see what may be amiss with the patient who is sitting before me. The next step is to *listen* – not always to what the patient has to say, but to the tone of their voice and breathing. At this point I also focus on the energies which vibrate from the body and the feedback I am getting. The next step is to *feel* all the pulses of the patient, their temperature

7

and to observe what problems, tangible and intangible, that patient might have.

I have a responsibility when a patient comes to me for help to find the problem, fix it and then leave it. I take a very sensible approach to the patient standing in front of me, wanting help. I look at them and ask myself the question, 'Where is the energy disturbed?' Life is energy and it is most important that it should be lived to the full. Even when the smallest part of the body is causing problems, help should be sought to restore that part because, in the short time that we are here, we want to get the most out of life.

It is most interesting how the tremendous field of energy that is in the body can be disturbed. It is equally interesting to see, when I use acupuncture, how with just one needle the blocked energy flow can be released and allowed to flow freely again, so that the vital force in the body will work effectively.

Just as a watchmaker has to know the location and function of the different mechanical parts in a watch as well as their names, the alternative health practitioner has to know the names of all the parts of the body, their location and function, and must have an expert understanding of the general principles of anatomy and physiology. We are all familiar with the common names of the organs and limbs. We know that the veins and arteries carry blood to every area, and that digestion is carried out in the abdominal area. We might even know the Latin names for even the most intricate parts of the body. It is important not just to memorise the anatomical names, but also to know what action needs to be taken when problems arise. It is essential for practitioners to look at the body as a whole and to study anatomy (which is interesting for nearly everybody), so that they will have knowledge that will allow them decide what treatments should be carried out to improve a patient's condition.

Looking at the human body as a machine, we see that it is composed of three parts. The first of these is the skeleton, made up of bones held together by ligaments, joints and muscles which introduce motion, nerves to control the action of the muscles, and blood vessels, which provide a source of nutrition and waste removal.

The second part of the body is the mind, a gift from God that makes us different from our fellow creatures. The third part is the extremely delicate processing and manufacturing plant which is contained within the body, the viscera. This processing plant is designed to take in a variety of raw materials and to convert them into products usable by the various components of the factory of the body. These three parts, whilst often separated by the manipulator, psychiatrist and physician respectfully, are actually part of one complete, functional unit, welded together by the autonomous nervous system.

The autonomous nervous system with its chemical counterpart, the endocrine system, constitutes the great two-way street by which the three major components of the human body are linked. Anything, large or small, which happens in one area will be reflected in one or both of the others. There is a general tendency in modern health practitioners to limit themselves to treating two parts of the body, the mind and the viscera, while ignoring the mechanical and electrical areas, but the three must always be considered as a whole.

Life means movement; perfect form means rhythmic balance. All humans are made up of atoms and it is this life force which maintains the normal rhythm of their bodies.

The nervous system controls every function of the body. If the motor system is disturbed, excessive or deficient physical action ensues; if the sensory system is disturbed, the result will be pain. The sympathetic nervous system is the superintendent of all the bodily functions. We must seek always to establish and improve the circulation of the blood and other fluids.

Interestingly, in Chinese medicine a great deal can be diagnosed from the skin. The layers of the skin are known as the epidermis and the derma, and there is also a third layer composed of fatty tissue, sometimes known as subcutaneous fat. The condition of the skin, the hair and the glands can give us a lot of information about what is taking place inside the body.

If we examine the anatomy and structure of the body, we see how it is composed, and this type of study includes all animal and plant life. The science of looking at the functions of the body, how it operates, is known as 'human physiology'. It is very important to learn as much about the body as possible, as we will come to discover in this book.

The body is basically divided into three parts – the head, the trunk and the extremities.

The head consists of a number of separate bones, fitted together as the skull, covered with muscles, flesh and skin. The head contains the eyes, the ears, the nose and the mouth. Inside and on top of this bony structure, we find the brain – the primary centre for regulating and coordinating body functions.

The trunk – which is the portion of the body exclusive of the head and the limbs – is divided into three sections: the chest, the abdomen and the pelvis. The chest (technically called the thorax), located between the base of the neck and the diaphragm, consists of the trachea, lungs, oesophagus, heart, circulatory system, pulmonary system, veins and arteries, aorta, pleura, vena cava, sternum, ribs and muscles, very intricately put together. The gullet (or oesophagus) is the tube that carries the food from the mouth to the stomach and includes the windpipe, which is technically known as the trachea. Below the thorax we find the large cavity called the abdominal cavity. This is separated from the thorax by a large wall of muscle. The abdominal cavity contains all the organs that are concerned with digestion: the stomach, the small intestine, the large intestine (known as the colon), the liver, the kidneys, the spleen, the gall bladder and the pancreas. In the lower part of the abdomen (called the pelvic region), we find the bladder and the rectum. The regenerative organs and sex organs are also found in the pelvic region.

The shoulder, arm, forearm and hand are known as the upper extremities; the thigh, leg and foot are the lower extremities. Thus, in anatomy, when we refer to the arm, we mean the upper part of the upper limb, being that portion of the upper extremities located between the elbow and the shoulder, and when we refer to the leg, we mean only the part of the lower limb located between the knee and ankle.

Now we will look at the most important part of the body – the cells. Cells are the building blocks from which every part of the body is formed. They are microscopic in size, so small that they cannot be seen with the naked eye, and are of various shapes and sizes, depending on their function. Each cell is a complex living unit in itself, able to digest food, take in oxygen, expel waste products and reproduce, with the exception of the nerve cells, which are totally different. The cell centre is called the nucleus. The central portion, where the cell reproduces itself and manufactures additional cells, is the protoplasm, and consists of various elements, such as carbon, iron and sodium, suspended in a thick, colourless liquid-like material containing a large amount of water. The entire cell is surrounded by the cell wall.

Up until the nineteenth century, very little was known about the nature of life. Since then we have discovered that life is the renewing of cell tissue and therefore cells may well be compared to bricks, joined together to form all the tissues and organs of the body, including the bones. Some of the cells have the special ability to feel cold, heat, pressure, etc. Together they make up the nervous system, which carries messages to and from the brain. The cells that are able to contract and expand are joined together to build muscles. The more commonly known cells are those found in the bloodstream, the red blood cells and the white blood cells.

The tissues consist of cells linked together to form a special fabric or structure in the body. There are various types of tissues – skin tissue, muscular tissue, connective tissue, cartilage tissue and nerve tissue – which we are all acquainted with. Tissue, and other cells, is massed together to form the organs. The eyes, ears, nose, tongue and skin are known as the sensory organs, providing us with the five senses. In my book, *The Five Senses*, I give a lot of information on seeing, hearing, smelling, tasting and feeling.

The body is divided into nine principal systems which are composed of tissues and organs, each having a specific function in its operation. These are:

- the vascular system
- the muscular system
- the nervous system
- the excretory system
- the respiratory system
- the alimentary system
- the skeletal system
- external secretions
- the reproductive system

This is a summarised version of the body. It is, however, much more complicated than that. When I look at a patient's whole system, I think of energy and where that may be disturbed. I am quite sure that the future of medicine is energy, so I want to go into great detail in this part of the book about the importance of harmonising it in the body where it has been disturbed.

To understand what being a doctor, surgeon, acupuncturist, manipulation therapist or even a patient really entails, we need

11

to know a little bit about how the body functions as a whole.

## BONES
The word skeleton is derived from the Greek word for 'mummy'. As many of the mummies, when found, consisted mostly of bones, anatomists applied the word to indicate the bony framework of the body. One of the important functions of the skeleton is to act as a protective covering for vital body organs, such as the brain, lungs and heart. Without this structure, the body would be a flabby shapeless mass incapable of any motion. Therefore, the skeleton acts as a framework for the body, as well as a means of locomotion. It also serves as a surface for the attachment of muscles and, as muscles by themselves can neither push nor pull, these movements are also dependent on the bones themselves, assisted by the muscles. A bone never moves on its own – it is the muscles that move it.

Bones are formed of cells and connective tissue. A large amount of lime salts (especially calcium phosphate) accumulate in and around the connective tissue cells in early life, making them rigid, with a stony hardness that permits them to withstand a lot of weight and pressure without bending or breaking. When we examine the bones, such as the clavicle, sternum, scapula, ribs and patella, the large bones, short bones, flat bones and irregular bones, it is quite astonishing to see how they all join together.

I deal with cartilage a lot in my work. It is found in every joint of the body, holds the skeleton together and is not only tough but also flexible and elastic. These properties are essential. In the spine there is a piece of cartilage between each vertebrae, known as the intervertebral cartilage. In addition to assisting the movement of the spine, this cartilage also act as a shock absorber.

The ribs are joined to the sternum (the breastbone) with cartilage, allowing a certain amount of movement, such as is needed when breathing or absorbing a sharp blow on the chest. The surfaces of bones that come into contact with other bones at the joints and sockets, where the bone articulates, are covered with cartilage. As cartilage is also formed of connective tissue and constantly replaces itself, it is of great assistance in preventing wear and assuring smooth movement in the joints.

The skeleton acts as support for the body and protects parts of it. The bones have two other very important functions. If we were to cut a bone – such as the femur – in half lengthwise and look inside, we would see that the outer layer of the bone consists of a very hard substance resembling ivory. The hollow central part consists of a soft pulpy substance called marrow, which is of two types, red and yellow. It is the red marrow in the bones that produces red and white blood corpuscles, as well as the blood platelets which are present in the proper proportion to other elements. The yellow marrow is a form of concentrated fatty material which can act as a form of chemical energy when nourishment is badly needed.

It is a fact that calcium is important to the blood and, actually, to every type of cell in the body. The bones are able to store it when there is an excess in the blood and if our body needs extra calcium, the blood can take it from this store.

## MUSCLES

Legend tells us that in ancient times, hunters observed that when a long muscle exposed in a living animal was tapped, a wave ran along the muscle, making it resemble a scurrying mouse. The word 'muscle' literally means 'little mouse'.

When the skin, which forms the external covering of the body, is removed, flesh known as lean meat is exposed. This flesh is actually the muscle tissue and is white in colour: it is the blood circulating through the muscle which gives it the red colouring associated with lean meat.

Wherever movement is needed, muscle tissue is found. It makes up 50 per cent of body weight in an athlete (due to the exercise and growth of the muscles) and approximately 40 per cent of body weight in other people. When it is realised that every movement of the body, including the beating of the heart and the digestion of food is dependent on muscle, there is no need to stress its importance in our daily life.

Muscles are formed of cells which have become elongated and developed into fibres. These fibres are held together in bundles with an intercellular substance which acts as a cement. The bundles are covered with a membrane called a 'muscle sheath' and groups of these membrane-covered fibres are held together, in turn, with an outside sheath, much as a group of rubber bands might be held together with elastic tape.

In addition to their function of articulating the skeleton, practically all body heat is supplied by the muscles. This heat is created by the muscles while changing form and pulling. The simple act of standing or sitting calls many muscles into play, creating heat. Part of the reason it is necessary to use covers when we go to bed at night is the smaller amount of heat produced when more of the muscles are at rest.

## THE NERVOUS SYSTEM

Of all the systems in the body, the nervous system may be considered as the master system and the nerve tissue the master tissue. Every organ in the body is dependent, in part, on the activity of some other organ. Muscular activity, for instance, requires additional respiration, heart action and circulation. A regulating power is needed to ensure that all the body systems are properly coordinated and work in harmony. This regulating power is the nervous system. It is composed of three parts:

- the central system
- the peripheral system
- the autonomic nervous system

The central and peripheral nervous systems are together known either as the cerebral spinal system or the voluntary nervous system. The central nervous system consists of the brain and the spinal cord. The brain, which is very soft and delicate and of vast importance to the whole body, is protected on the outside by solid bone covering the skull. The divisions of the brain are: the cerebrum, the cerebellum, the midbrain, the pons Varolli and the medulla oblongata.

## THE CIRCULATORY SYSTEM

The circulatory system of the body has many duties to perform, such as the carrying of nutrition to all the cells, oxygen from the lungs and digested food from the intestines. It also assists in the elimination of waste products from the cells. There are approximately nine pints of blood in the circulatory system of the average person and it is very important that this blood is kept in constant circulation in order that it may cover every portion of the body and perform its normal function.

The blood vascular system is classified as:

- the circulatory medium blood
- the heart
- the blood vessels
- the regulating mechanism

## THE LYMPHATIC SYSTEM

One of the most important systems in the body is the lymphatic system. Unfortunately, there are often a lot of problems with it. It is a circulatory system with which most people are not familiar, transporting a fluid called lymph around the body. Unlike the blood vascular system, the lymphatic system does not have a heart to use as a propelling force – it is dependent on the movements of the muscles and joints for its propulsion through the body. The lymphatic system consists of lymph fluid, lymphatic vessels through which the lymph flows, lymph nodes and a large organ called the spleen. You will find it interesting to see in some of the case histories in this book how often the lymphatic system plays a part in twenty-first-century diseases.

I often think of my great friend and teacher, the American naturopath Dr Leonard Allan, who said, 'Life is energy and energy is life.'

## THE HEAD

### Parts of the Skull

Although there is little that can be directly accomplished with massage where the bones of the skull are concerned, they are indirectly benefited by massage of the head, due to the stimulation of nerves and the activation of the blood supply that nourishes the bones.

The skull rests upon the spinal column, and has been divided by anatomists for the purpose of study into two main sections – the cranium (containing the brain – also known as the 'brain case') and the face (or anterior region).

#### The Bones of the Cranium

The cranium is formed by the following bones: the occipital, parietal, frontal, temporal, ethmoid and sphenoid.

##### The Occipital Bone

The occipital bone derives its name from a Latin word indicating the back of the head. The occipital bone, therefore, is found at the base of the skull, and helps to form the 'floor' of the cranium. There is a large foramen (opening) in the lower portion of the occipital bone, through which the medulla oblongata passes, to join the spinal cord. The occipital bone also has two processes called condyles, which are shaped like flattened knobs, and which articulate (form a joint) with the atlas (the first spinal bone).

*The Parietal Bones*
The parietal bone derives its name from a Latin word meaning 'wall'. There are two parietal bones, one on each side of the skull. Meeting in the centre, they form the main wall of the cranium or skull.

*The Frontal Bone*
The frontal bone forms the forehead and the roof of the sockets for the eyes (orbital cavities). In the inner angle of the orbital cavities, there are two small depressions in the frontal bone in which the lacrimal glands (tear ducts) are set. These are the ducts that keep the eyes moist by constantly washing them.

*The Temporal Bones*
There are two temporal bones, one on each side of the skull in the region of the ears. They derive their name from a Latin word meaning 'time', as it was found that the hair first begins to turn grey in this area, thus indicating the passing of time. The temporal bones contain two very important structures. One of these, at the bottom of the temporal bone, is the opening to the middle ear (that part of the ear in which vibrations are carried to the brain). The other structure is the mastoid process, which is the part of the bone that goes down behind the lower part of the ear. The mastoid portion of the temporal bone is in the form of a honeycomb. The cavities are called mastoid cells, or sinuses. These contain air and have an opening to the cavity of the middle ear. Inflammation of the lining of these mastoid cells results in the condition known as mastoiditis. There is also a slender, pointed piece of bone which goes downward from the under surface of the temporal bone, called the styloid process, to which are attached some of the muscles of the tongue.

*The Ethmoid Bone*
The ethmoid bone derives its name from a Greek word meaning 'sieve', and is a small, irregular mass of spongy bone of no particular shape. The ethmoid bone is found in the nasal cavity. It has numerous perforations through which the olfactory nerves (nerves of smell) pass, going to the nose.

### The Sphenoid Bone

The sphenoid bone derives its name from a Latin word meaning 'wedge'. The body of the sphenoid bone has two broad wing-like processes which help to form the frontal part of the cranial cavity. The centre of the sphenoid sags down, forming a saddle-like depression, in which some of the glands found in the head are located. The lower part of the wing-like process of the sphenoid acts as the origin of the muscles found in the palate.

## The Bones of the Face

The features of the face are formed by the following bones: the nasal, zygomatic, maxilla and mandible.

### The Nasal Bones

The nasal bones are two small bones set in the middle and upper part of the face, and form the bridge or upper part of the nose (the lower part of the nose is formed entirely of cartilage).

### The Zygomatic Bones

The zygomatic bones take their name from a Greek word meaning 'cheekbones'. The zygomatic bones form the lower outer half of the orbital cavity (eye sockets) and go towards the back of the head as a long, narrow bone, known as the temporal process, which articulates with the temporal bone. The zygomatic bones can be felt as the prominences on each side of the face, known as the cheekbones.

### The Maxilla Bones

There are two maxilla bones and they derive their name from a Latin word meaning 'jawbone'. They are aptly named, in that they form the upper jaw. The maxilla form the lower, inner half of the orbital cavity, the opening for the nose, and the greater part of the roof of the mouth. Each bone has a spongy margin which is the base on which the upper teeth are fitted. In the region of the cheeks, the maxilla are hollow, thus forming a sinus (or cavity), which opens in the nose.

### The Mandible Bone

The mandible bone, or lower jaw, derives its name from a Latin word meaning 'jaw'. It also has a soft, spongy recess in which the lower teeth are set. The lower jawbone is notched on each side. The back part of the notch is called the condyle, and fits into a depression in the temporal bone for the purpose of articulation. The front part of the notch, called the coronoid process, serves as the seat of origin for some of the facial muscles. The mandible goes up at a sharp angle called the 'oblique line' on top, and the 'angle' underneath. The mandible is the largest and strongest bone in the face and is the bone that performs all of the movements when chewing, the upper jaw being stationary.

### The Foramen
The word foramen is derived from a Latin word meaning 'opening'. On the bones of the face these foramen serve as openings through which nerves and blood vessels pass, and thus come in contact with either the inside or outside of a bone area, as the case may be, in order to provide proper blood and nerve supply. The mental foramen allows the passage of a dental nerve, supplying the molar teeth of the lower jaw; therefore, when applying massage in this area, you are actually stimulating the nerve that supplies these teeth.

## BLOOD VASCULAR SYSTEM OF THE HEAD

### The Common Carotid Arteries
There are two common carotid arteries and these derive their name from a Greek word meaning 'deep sleep'. It has been found that deep pressure on these arteries produces anaemia of the brain, resulting in unconsciousness. The left common carotid branches from the upper surface of the arch of the aorta. The right common carotid forms at the division of the innominate artery. In the neck (in the region of the thyroid cartilage, or Adam's apple), the common carotid arteries divide into two branches called the 'internal' and 'external' carotid arteries.

#### The External Carotid Artery
Upon branching off from the common carotid artery, the external carotid artery continues up the neck, forming numerous branches that cover the neck, face and scalp. Each carotid artery covers its own side of the face: that found on the left side covers the whole of that side of the head, whereas that on the right side of the neck covers the right side of the head. The external carotid arteries furnish the blood supply to the thyroid gland, tongue, throat, face and ears, as well as the dura mater inside the cranium.

*The Internal Carotid Artery*
This artery, upon leaving the common carotid, goes deeper into the neck than the external carotid, finally entering the cranial cavity (the base of the skull containing the brain, through a small opening or foramen called the 'carotid canal'). In the cranium, the internal carotid finally branches off, forming arteries which supply the brain and the eyes.

The common carotid arteries, with the branches they form, are responsible for the distribution of the blood supply to the brain, as well as to the rest of the head.

### The Vertebral Arteries
The vertebral arteries assist the internal carotid to supply the brain with fresh blood. These arteries are branches of the subclavian arteries that are found on the two sides of the body in the region of the shoulders. The vertebral arteries, branching off from the subclavian, run towards the back of the neck, where they enter the foramen in the transverse process of the cervical vertebrae and, going upward, enter the cranial cavity. In the cranial cavity, the vertebral arteries give off a pair of arteries to feed the cerebellum, then unite to form a single artery called the 'basilar artery'.

### The Basilar Artery
The basilar artery, having been formed by the uniting of two vertebral arteries, then separates and forms two arteries called the 'posterior (to the rear) cerebral arteries', each of which, in turn, divide and send a branch to unite with the internal carotid artery. These vessels cover and supply the entire base of the brain with fresh arterial blood.

## VEINS OF THE HEAD AND NECK
The arteries in the head, forming smaller and smaller arteries, finally form capillaries. These, in turn, form the veins that drain the toxic blood from the head. The veins, growing larger, unite with each other, in much the same fashion as small streams, flowing into each other, form larger streams. Thus, the small veins growing larger and larger finally form the 'jugular veins'.

### The Jugular Veins
It is understood by most people that there is a jugular vein in the neck. However, very few laymen realise that the neck has four

jugular veins, with one external and one internal jugular vein being found on each side of the neck.

### The Internal Jugular Veins

The two internal jugular veins are formed inside the cranium by the many small veins that drain the area of the brain and pass out of the cranium into the neck, through two openings called the 'jugular foramen'. On their way down the sides of the neck, the internal jugular veins receive the flow of many smaller veins that drain the face and neck. At the base of the neck, the internal jugular veins unite with the subclavian veins, which come up from the arms, and thus form the right and left innominate veins.

### The External Jugular Veins

The external jugular veins are closer to the surface of the neck than the internal jugular veins, and also smaller in size. Many of the veins of the face and neck unite to form the external jugular veins. These external jugular veins, in turn, pour the toxic blood they carry into the subclavian veins.

## MUSCLES OF THE HEAD

### The Epicranial Muscle

The epicranial muscle, also known as the 'occipital frontalis', may be considered two muscles – the occipital, covering the back part of the skull, and the frontalis, covering the front of the skull. The occipital and frontalis are held together in the centre of the skull by a thin aponeurosis (part of the connective tissue covering the top of the cranium that forms a ridge in the centre of the head, where the muscles are attached to it).

The occipital muscle originates at the occipital bone and the mastoid portion of the temporal bone (behind the lower part of the ear), and inserts into the aponeurosis in the centre of the head. The frontal muscle originates from the aponeurosis and inserts into the tissue over the eyes.

The frontal part of the epicranial muscle is the more powerful. It is used in elevating the eyebrows, thus causing the skin of the forehead to fold into lines or wrinkles. The occipital muscle simply draws the scalp backwards.

## MUSCLES OF THE FACE
There are over 30 muscles in the face. However, only those of primary interest in the field of massage will be described here.

### The Orbicularis Oculi
The orbicularis oculi is a muscle that derives its name from a Latin word meaning 'little circle surrounding the eye'. The orbicularis oculi originates from the nasal portion of the frontal bone (the short bone forming the upper part of the nose), and the frontal process of the maxilla (the upper jaw), close to the side of the nose. It spreads into a broad, thin layer that covers the eyelid and inserts at the union of the upper and lower lid on the outer corner of the eye. The second portion of the orbicularis oculi surrounds the orbit (the opening in the skull that holds the eye), spreading onto the temple and downward on the cheek, thus forming a complete circle of the orbital cavity. The orbicularis oculi closes the eyelid gently when sleeping or blinking. It also assists in tightening the brow.

### The Orbicularis Oris
The orbicularis oris takes its name from a Latin word meaning 'little circle surrounding the mouth'. This muscle consists of fibres that are derived from other muscles, which all unite to form a circular muscle that surrounds and inserts in the lips. Other small muscles, in turn, insert in the orbicularis oris at the corners of the mouth to assist in pulling the corners of the mouth in various directions, such as bringing them up in smiling, or down when scowling. The orbicularis oris compresses the lips against the teeth, or causes them to protrude when pouting.

### The Buccinator Muscle
The buccinator, taken from the Latin word meaning 'trumpeter', is the muscle found on the cheeks. It originates from the maxilla and the mandible, and goes forward to insert at the sides of the mouth. It pulls the corners of the mouth back in a straight line and flattens the cheeks when the lips are closed.

### The Muscles of Mastication
The muscles that are involved in chewing are the following: the temporal, the masseter, and the external and internal pterygoid.

### The Temporal Muscle

The temporal muscle originates from the temporal region of the skull, passing downward past the zygomatic arch to insert in the mandible. Its function is to assist in closing the jaw.

### The Masseter Muscle

The masseter muscle originates at the zygomatic arch, and inserts on the upper part of the mandible, that section called the 'ramus'.

### The External and Internal Pterygoid Muscles

These muscles originate on the lower surface of the skull, and insert on the surface of the mandible, at the ramus. The internal pterygoid assists in closing the jaws, while the external pterygoid helps to open them. The moving of the jaws from side to side is the work of the pterygoid muscles. They produce this movement by exerting alternate pulling motions. When acting together, the pterygoid muscles protrude the jaw (pull it forward). The pterygoid muscles are found beneath the masseter and buccinator.

### The Platysma

The platysma has been named after a Greek word meaning 'plate'. It is a broad sheet-like muscle that originates from the skin and fascia (muscle covering) of the pectoral and deltoid muscles of the chest, climbing up the neck to insert at the mandible and muscles at the corner of the mouth. Its function is to depress the mandible (lower the jaw) and draw down the lower lip.

### The Sternocleidomastoid Muscle

The sternocleidomastoid muscle has a complicated name. However, it was named after the locations of its origin and insertion. It originates in two parts, from the upper part of the sternum and the inner border of the clavicle (the breastbone), then unites to go up the neck to insert by a strong tendon into the mastoid section of the temporal bone. This muscle can be seen easily on thin people, as it is the one that gives a cord-like appearance to each side of the neck. It can also be seen to protrude along each side of the neck when the head is turned sharply in the opposite direction.

The two sternocleidomastoid muscles, when acting together,

pull the head forward and, when taking a deep breath, assist in lifting the thorax (chest). When one muscle acts alone, it draws the head towards the shoulder on the side of its insertion.

Having studied the anatomy of the face, you should now realise how, by activating and bringing tone to the muscles of the face, you can assist in the treatment of many facial conditions, such as torticollis, or wry-neck, facial spasm, sagging muscles which distort the face, and numerous other conditions.

It is best to keep in mind that in massage, you are not simply working on the surface of the body, but are activating muscles, tissues and the venous circulation lying below the surface, and also stimulating nerves. Therefore, it is necessary that you have some knowledge of what lies beneath the skin in the area upon which you are applying massage, in order to give a professional treatment.

## RULES FOR HEALTH AND HEALING

1. Remote pain is never in the bone, but always in the tissue.
2. Polarity is the law governing the relativity of all being – the positive, negative and the neutral.
3. We provide the mould for the creative law and unless the mould is increased, the substance cannot increase.
4. Man is fundamentally made perfect – always separate the disease from the person suffering with it. Disease has no location, no expression. Never locate a disease, because thoughts are things and if given power, will begin to operate.
5. Be specific in treating, be definite and direct in your mental work. You are dealing with intelligence, so deal with it intelligently. Anyone can heal themselves who believes they can, if they will take the time to put that belief into motion.
6. Every time we think, we are thinking into a receptive, plastic substance which receives the impression of our thoughts. When we stop to realise how subtle thoughts are, how we unconsciously think negatively and how easy it is to become down, we see that everyone perpetuates their own condition. That is why people go from bad to worse and from success to great success.
7. All diseases have one common origin and that origin is a toxic condition resulting from food fermentation. This

has a great influence upon the condition of a patient, although symptoms are frequently looked at and treated as the cause. A fast can often cure a disorder, for the simple reason that fasting gives the cells of the body a chance to get rid of toxins.

8. Within everyone is a force which directs and controls the entire course of their lives. It can heal every affliction and ailment.

9. All attempts at healing, regardless of the medium through which they are made, are, in reality, attempts to regulate and re-establish the normal rhythm (or energy) of the body.

10. Energy must flow. Any sore spots are blocks in the energy current at either the positive, negative or neutral poles. One must locate where the energy block exists before it can be released. When the balance is re-established, the pain will leave at once and normal activity will take place.

## MAGNETIC FIELDS

In dealing with the body's magnetic fields, whether it be for diagnosis or for treatment, the north–south position is very important for the positive, long axis of the body. The east–west position is just as important for the circular axis, or the magnetic waves around the long axis. In healing, if possible, it is better for patients to be placed with their heads facing to the north in order to benefit from this positive axis. Healing depends on this and local polarisation of the patient's own energy fields, achieved by releasing spasms which are usually located in the sympathetic nervous system.

When anything in life changes its frequency from normal and ceases to move, it dies.

The perineal technique balances the energy fields, acting on the circulation and relieving spasticity or congestion.

## THE HUMAN BODY AND MAGNETIC FIELDS

There are billions of cells in every square inch of tissue in the human body. It is a scientific fact that every one of these cells has an inbuilt intelligence. The cells breathe and excrete waste matter and can even live independently of the human body, indefinitely.

When the Creator gave us our perfect body, he also gave us a complete set of controls to keep it in perfect order and harmony.

Viruses and germs do not cause our aches and pains or our deficiencies and infections. They can never really harm a body that is in a healthy state, a balanced creation of physical, mental and spiritual attributes.

It was once said by a great philosopher, Hermes, that 'Everything flows out and in. Everything has its tides. All things rise and fall; rhythm compensates.' The very same principle manifests itself in the positive, negative and neutral energies of the body, even when we go through the necessary process of breathing.

It is very difficult to understand exactly how these energies work. In China, as I have said, I learned to look, listen and feel. Once I have done this with a patient, I go on to look at their body as a field of energy and aim to balance positive and negative, the left side of the body being negative and the right positive. One can sometimes do this very easily. Many years ago my eldest daughter, who was nursing in a London hospital at the time, told me of a Japanese professor who worked there using copper and zinc magnets, and who was holding a seminar. I thought his technique was probably just a gimmick but I wanted to go, especially because it was being held in one of the hospitals. Many doctors were present. It was quite amazing to see how this professor, with the use of copper and zinc magnets, balanced energies in patients. After he had placed the magnets on the sacrum, in opposite directions, it was possible to see the sacrum almost pulling itself into balance, if one of the legs had been longer or shorter than the other.

One can also do a lot with one's hands, and as the Americans often say, the thumb is very important when undertaking reflexology or aromatherapy. It can be used as a neutral to balance positive and negative. This might sound complicated, but it is actually very simple. Nowadays, many practitioners use magnetic therapy as part of their treatment. It also has the added advantage that patients can self-administer the therapy to great effect. There are also special courses available in this field and the results that can be achieved through it are tremendous.

The heart centre is the pivot for the circulation of these energies in the blood. Through it, it becomes the control centre for the body's vital force. Contact with the positive right hand with the neutral thumb over the heart, at the same time as the negative-energy left hand is placed anywhere on the body that needs healing, can do much to alleviate pains where there are energy blocks in the circulation.

The diaphragm is one of the most important organs in the whole of the human body. The action of the diaphragm occasioned by proper breathing causes an internal massage of the vital organs of digestion. This type of breathing can be learned in yoga. The good breather is unlikely to suffer from liver troubles, spleen or pancreas dysfunction, for the motion of the diaphragm tends to keep these organs in a good state of health. Freeing the diaphragm by contact with the hands under the floating ribs on both sides and under the sternum is a very important technique for releasing blocks in the bloodstream.

Remember that no one magnetic pole dominates the body over the others. If the treatment of the negative pole alone refuses to give the desired results, the patient should not feel disheartened.

The therapist's right hand should always be on the most negative pole (the toes), the left hand on the neutral pole (the fingers), in the middle or on the neck or head (positive), if the current stimulated is strong enough to carry that far. If not, go a little above the lowest contact and establish a current between the two hands by kneading and pressing them, then proceed in this manner up to the neutral centre pole, then on to the neck and head, the positive pole, above.

Disease usually manifests itself in three areas: the top, the middle and the bottom. In this form of therapy, acute and painful conditions are usually treated in the same direction as the current flow, which tends to be from above downwards. All chronic and abnormal conditions are treated by beginning at the extremities and working in an inward and upward direction. Often, a heat lamp shone on the patient's bare feet is a boon and a great help in stimulating the current flow to the lowest point or extremity. The feet and toes are the extremities of the negative pole in the current flow and it is there that most energy blocks are formed. Releasing these blocks is very important. The hands are the neutral poles of the human body.

Respiration is closely connected with the emotional impulses and the heartbeat. The diaphragm is the respiratory muscle and the right and left phrenic nerve supply this muscle. The negative pole of the heart's sensory centre is located in the perineal floor. These muscles synchronise with the diaphragm in respiration. The occiput forms the positive pole of a broad triangular space which covers the motor area and centres of involuntary function.

There are a few points to note while we are on the subject of polarity. The temporal bone is the positive pole of the innominates. The rectal sphincter and gullet respond to each other as positive and negative areas. The anterior sphincter has a reflex to the throat (dryness, coughing, tickling in the throat). The sacrum is the negative pole to the brain, the pituitary is the positive pole. Write that down in your brain and remember it. The sphenoid is the positive pole (the ganglion of Rebes); the coccyx is the negative pole (the ganglion of Impar). The specific polarity reflex in the neck is of the neutral pole of the hands between the thumbs and first fingers.

Every source of power – electricity, fuel, minerals, vegetable or animal – is only a manifestation of another phase of gravity. Living cells are self-changing condensers built on the fundamental plan of the atom and the molecule. Electricity is the thread which binds together form and function.

All living matter has what we call a life force. It is this which distinguishes living forms. The mystery of life is really the mystery of why and how a living cell, materially similar in every respect to a non-living cell, can continually discharge energy – that is, continue to carry on the evidence of life.

There is a reciprocal action between positive and negative charges of electricity in the atom, molecule and cell, and also in the animal. In all living organisms some cells are more positive in reaction than others. These cells form the positive pole of the body in the brain cells. The liver is the negative pole of the body, collecting the waste products, since the negative pole of any electrical circuit collects the waste. The cell, and in fact the body as a whole, operates on the same principle and has the same function as an electric battery.

The centre of gravity in the human body is roughly one inch headward from the sacrum. This is a fundamental loose link that proves the fact that no structure is distorted until the centre of gravity is displaced.

Seeming miracles can be brought about with polarity balance. The muscles are first relaxed and freed from spasm, enabling fresh blood to permeate the stagnant tissues. Always remember that the sympathetic nervous system sends to every part of the body the curative, creative, repairing energy that cures diseases and repairs injuries. Energy in the three nervous systems flows like an electrical current with a vibratory nature and has the triune quality of negative, positive and neutral. The energy used by the sympathetic nervous system is always of a creative, constructive and healing nature. It carries and distributes to all parts of the body a vital, intangible energy that vitalises the organs and cells of the body and gives them new energy and a lift.

A fuller study of the autonomous nervous system would also pay dividends.

## HEALING AND HEALTH

In every analysis of disease and its cause it can be seen that there are three very important fundamental errors in the modern way of living:

1. Not eating the right foods to give the proper chemical balance in the body.
2. Not drinking half or even a third enough water each day to give the right amount of moisture in the body.
3. Not acting, exercising or living in a way that would assist the body to rid itself of the proper amount of waste matter each day. There is only one disease, physical or mental, and its name is Congestion.

True healing involves the harmonious relationship of the inner energies and outer energies. This factor has not yet been fully understood, nor has it been applied to its fullest extent. A new viewpoint and emphasis is needed in healthcare, to help improve the effectiveness of the body's energy fields and their structural balance with the earth's gravity and energies. Most of us should endeavour to understand the mystery of human life and the universe in which we live, move, breathe and have our being. Some of us realise, in a vague sort of way, that we are linked to Mother Nature and dependent on her forces for our existence. If we were to think impartially, especially with regards to the deeper problems of life, we would act to the best of our ability to change things for the better, and then we could sit back and wait for the results to speak for themselves. All human beings seem to be so frail and changeable in their understanding of the great truths and even seem averse to applying these truths or researching them.

Healing is akin to electricity – one cannot define it or interpret it but its action can not only be seen, but felt as well. The human body is in a state of flux all the time because, without the expansion and contraction of all the body tissues, there would be no life at all. We will learn, as we proceed, how we can alter these fluctuations and use them for healing purposes.

Much has been written on the many facets of the healing arts. There are chiropractors, osteopaths, mechano-therapists and many more. The list of all the types of therapist alone would fill many pages. Please remember that all these practitioners do very valuable work in relieving the sufferings of the afflicted. They could do still more, however, if they applied the natural laws governing health. These laws are immutable and many suffer when they endeavour to change them even an iota. On the other hand, better health will be found when these immutable laws are applied to life and living.

Pain is one of the main manifestations of disease to drive patients to the clinic for treatment. All of us want and seek the relief of pain desperately, yet pain should be our friend, as it is the only way our body knows of telling us that there is danger ahead. It stops us in our path and makes us think about ourselves. Before we can really call ourselves health practitioners, we must delve further into the cause of the pain, as all physical troubles begin and end in pain.

Pain is a sensory perception. It is a partial break in the circuit of the centripetal energy flow in the nervous system. Health is a balance between contraction and over-relaxation. Most pains are the product of over-contraction. Contraction usually results in acidosis, relaxation results in alkalinity. The balance between contraction and relaxation is a very fine one. Contraction is usually an effect of the sympathetic nervous system and expansion is an effect of the parasympathetic nervous system. Inflammation and pain is the tissue response to injury. Pain is really an instrument that helps us realise when we need treatment and when we don't.

If you made life into an equation, it would appear as follows:

HEALTH     =     Environment     =     ADAPTATION
                 Resistance

Dr Carrell wrote in his book, *Man The Unknown*,

> Through his nervous system, man records the stimuli
> impinging upon him from his environment. His organs
> and muscles supply the appropriate lever. He struggles
> for existence with his mind, even more than with his
> body, to make the right decision.

It is now an established fact that the sympathetic nervous system holds the key to health and all therapies are subservient to this. The public today want fast relief, and are not in the slightest interested in healthy eating or hearing lectures on nature's laws. Unfortunately, they do not want to know and their only immediate interest is for you to get them out of the quagmire of ill health.

The healing of the future will be based on the atom, within and without the body. A bone moved by mechanical means will not stay put for long, and never permanently, unless the cause is attended to first. It is the ligaments and tendons that move muscles which, in turn, move bones out of alignment. But what is the cause? All muscles contract and expand naturally. When this is done too rapidly, a spasm and pain result.

Every molecule and every atom in the universe, animate and inanimate, is in constant vibration. Each mineral and each life cell in man, animal or insect, vibrates on its own frequency and wavelength. Also, there are vibrations of sound, of colour, and of smell, of heat and of light. In addition, the earth and all its living things are continuously being bombarded by stellar vibrations and cosmic rays of a frequency too high for us to comprehend. Furthermore, the earth is surrounded and criss-crossed by magnetic bands, man-made radio currents, all vibratory in nature. These are facts, governed by natural law.

Vibrations of sound can cause pleasure or pain, according to their effect on our emotions. A rhythmic tune will start our feet tapping involuntarily, while a plaintive melody will often bring a lump to the throat and cause tears. A dog will yelp in pain at the blast of a whistle and howl mournfully at the strains of a violin. There is also power in the human voice, to influence or offend. The ancient people knew of the power of the spoken word – an old proverb says, 'A soft answer turneth away wrath'.

Most powerful of all, but least understood, are the cosmic vibrations. There can be no doubt that they exercise a profound influence on our lives. We are in constant contact with the heavenly forces that radiate through our body and these forces, in their descent through us to earth, make us into living human magnets. Our arms and hands are true extensions of this constant, powerful cosmic energy. Our feet should be in firm contact with Mother Earth. It's up to us to harness and use these forces to help ourselves and our fellow human beings. Humans are complete entities: body, mind and soul.

It is a very well-known fact that as long as we learn from life and forget ourselves, we are growing and living. All life is like a song — it has its own rhythm of harmony, it is a symphony of all things which exist in major and minor keys of polarity. It can blend the discord caused by opposites into a harmony which unites the whole. Any limitations we have are products of our own thinking. The moulds of pleasure, of pain, health and sickness etc. are formed by our own thoughts and its patterns of harmony and discord.

The ancient Chinese found methods of balancing the body and its polarities. They are still being applied today by many different schools. They believed that there were two forms of energy (or Chi): positive (yang) and negative (yin). It must be realised that all things in their whole beings are of a triune nature, the centre of these energies being the neutral, from which come the positive and then the negative. All things must have a centre, like a stick, which has two ends but also a centre, which is neutral. Take a bar magnet. It has a positive pole and a negative, but at the centre there is a neutral area. When we understand and apply these forces, we will be able to heal the sick in accordance with nature's law. All matter is composed of vibrating energy and must have positive, negative and neutral forces within, in order to make a complete whole. The balance of the three is the healing of the future and is an active factor in the process of all creation.

It is agreed and well understood by scientists that humans have a physical body of solid and semi-solid matter, analysed by physiological, structural, mechanical, chemical, thermal, electrical, psychological and bacteriological fields of science. If that were all we consisted of, however, there would be no unfamiliar health problems or disease to torment those of us who endeavour to solve such problems daily.

There exists a vital form of life which is superior to and of a much finer substance than the physical. It is also independent of the grosser physical form. The gross body is made of two energy pattern fields, or halves. The right half of the body is positive and the left half of the body is negative. The upper part of the body, above the diaphragm, contains the positive element and the lower half of the body, below the diaphragm, contains the negative. The positive element gives warmth and energy. The diaphragm separates the above from the below and is the neutral field. The lower, or negative, part of the body

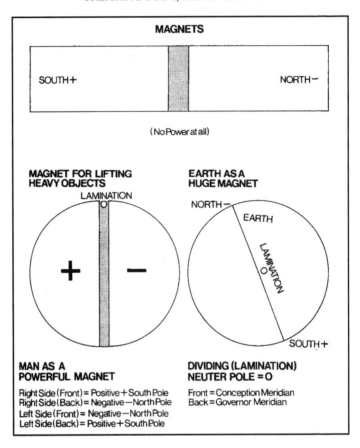

MAGNETS

SOUTH+    NORTH—

(No Power at all)

MAGNET FOR LIFTING
HEAVY OBJECTS
LAMINATION

+    —

EARTH AS A
HUGE MAGNET
NORTH—
EARTH
LAMINATION
O
SOUTH+

MAN AS A
POWERFUL MAGNET
Right Side (Front) = Positive + South Pole
Right Side (Back) = Negative —North Pole
Left Side (Front) = Negative —North Pole
Left Side (Back) = Positive + South Pole

DIVIDING (LAMINATION)
NEUTER POLE = O
Front = Conception Meridian
Back = Governor Meridian

nourishes the body, the pelvis being the negative pole.

The vital life force flows through all these energy fields and polarises them into active function. The ancients clearly understood that it was this life force (chi energy), which enters the body through one's breathing, that animates and controls the gross physical body functions.

The physical body is negative, while the vital body (the soul) is positive. The mental body is neutral, and can affect the whole because it is the central core of all the fields of the body. Just as the vital body blends with the physical in every cell, function and structure, the mental body penetrates every tissue cell of the entire body in normal health. A well-known axiom and immutable natural law is that 'Life proceeds from within outwards and from above downwards'. The three bodies are created firstly in fine patterns of mind energy, then in less intense currents of vital force, and finally in the gross body and its related energy fields of action.

In dealing with personal problems of mind and matter, especially in health and healing, we seem to have forgotten the basic principle upon which all matter, in all its manifestations, rests. Cause and effect is the law of motion. Two ends, a middle or a centre, and a circumference geometrically depict polarity. The foundation of my research into this is the simple concept that there are five fields of matter, five senses and five motor currents going over these fields in three modes of motion: positive, negative and neutral. Keep this in mind and a whole new concept of healing is possible. I have researched the principles of the triune essence and energy in all created things. It is energy in motion, expression and sensation. All energy must have a centre to move from and an objective to go to. The positive flow is outwards and is expressed as motor currents, whilst the return flow is negative and is expressed as sensory currents. The source, or reserve, of this energy lies in the centre (neutral), the nucleus from which it flows and to which it returns. The source of all energy is the internal neutral centre, around which the currents flow like the protons and electrons around a neutron. It is quite amazing to see how relaxed some patients become when they put their left hand on the tummy (under the navel) and the right hand on top of it, forming a magnetic force. If they then breath in through the nose, deep into the tummy, and out through the mouth, the energies harmonise themselves. This is a very important relaxation exercise. Energy in motion must have this triple action in order to function.

Polarity is the law of the finer relationships of everything in nature. It is the principle of attraction and repulsion in every area of life. Sensation in itself depends wholly on polarity; pleasure and pain are sensation's binary forces. Every sensation, action and impulse comes down in its most basic form to polarity impulse. Polarity is either attraction (pleasurable, sensory, ingoing energy) or repulsion (pain, or an outgoing force of action). The latter depends on tension and contraction, which are closely linked to pain. We have three bodies, the physical, the emotional and the mental.

We express energy every second. For every inhalation, there must be an exhalation, or the correct sequence of the polarity principle is broken. Short-circuits in the body must be found and restored before health can return.

Structural polarisation by means of current flow is an important factor in health. Fields become obstructed by gross matter, like the muscle tissue by carbon and acid deposits as well as other waste products. Mind always repels the grosser and attracts the finer forces and uses these as building blocks. In severe illness, there is a lack of active energy or life force. The brachial plexus is important, as it is the motor respiratory centre which governs the function of polarity. The sicker a patient, the more his or her shoulder blades will constrict the ribs. The brachial plexus is the main spring of the triune energies in action, for no respiration means no life, no motion. The brachial plexus governs the life force and is in fact the vital centre of life. It is more easily accessible to the practitioner from under the shoulder blades than at the spinal centres. Releasing tension in the sensory field by lifting the scapula is like giving wings to a bird. The finest therapy is that which balances the forces in a particular individual, not only in gross anatomy but also in the finer fields of the body's energies. When the root cause of a disease is found and properly treated, health and well-being will return.

## THE BODY'S CELLS

Each body cell is composed of atoms, is bipolar, has a nucleus of solar electricity and is dominated by magnetic force. The polar properties of attraction and repulsion are very marked in the cells. They unite and separate exactly as do two electrified bodies and that is what they are. Two other functions are expressed by the cell: volition and sensation. Volition is the power of selection and rejection. Sensation is the power of response or sensitiveness to impressions.

These four fundamental functions of the cell result from the action of solar forces on the poles of the cells, producing all phenomena summed up in the word 'life', with each organ and gland performing its allotted work. And there, right under the very nose of the scientist, we have Carrell's 'unknowable reality', Osler's expression of 'a series of chemical changes', Spencer's 'continuous adjustment of internal relations to external relations' and Bichat's 'sum of the functions [of the body] by which death is resisted'. There is that mysterious 'life principle' which scientists are unable to find or define, because they do not know what they are searching for.

Imagine an upright bar with negative and positive poles. To this, affix a crossbar with volition and sensation poles. Here we have the Cross of Life mentioned even by ancient nations long ago. This cross presents a clear picture of the four phases of solar electricity in relation to the human body and as manifested as vital force.

Creative processes also present these four fundamental functions inherent in the atom, which appear in the body cells in the form termed life.

## THE HUMAN ENIGMA

'God took to himself the dust of the earth and from it he made man; he then breathed into his nostrils the breath of life and man became a living soul.'

Humans seem to be the only creatures who are not aware of what they are doing or where they are going. Even the ants and the bees have an advance knowledge of the part they are destined to play in their lives.

We lack knowledge of the physiology of the nervous cells, how the mind is influenced by the state of the organs. Leave it to humans to get their priorities wrong; mystical laws became known long before those of physiology.

There is a reason for the slow progress of self-knowledge. The ancient way of life, co-habiting in small groups, has been replaced today by a herd mentality. Solitude is looked upon as a punishment, and sometimes as a luxury. Modern civilisation seems incapable of producing people endowed with imagination, intelligence and courage. Discoveries are developed without any foreknowledge of their consequences. Actually, we are becoming strangers in our own world. There is a possible remedy for this evil and it rests in a more profound knowledge of ourselves. The science of man has become the most necessary of all sciences.

'Man is a being composed of matter and consciousness.' Such a proposition is really meaningless. Every body is animated by an invisible power and this makes our physical beings possess the qualities of a magnet.

It is of no ultimate use for us to increase the comfort, the luxury, the beauty and the complications of our civilisation. All this will prove of no value if our weaknesses prevent us using our knowledge to our best advantage. Developing the study of our own body and nature will, and must, be the task of the future.

Soul and body are creations of our methods of observation. The human body is far too complex for us to comprehend in its entirety. The quality of any individual partly depends on that of their surface, as the brain is continually being moulded by the messages it receives from the outer world.

It behoves all of us to remember one thing: 'know thyself'.

He who has health has hope.
He who has hope has everything.

The ancient masters taught their disciples how to control the vibrations of the pituitary and pineal glands, the glands of the sixth and seventh sense powers, in a manner that enabled them to contact any region of the inner worlds that they desired to visit, as we do in dreams when we sleep.

I repeat, the body must have three poles of energy: the positive, the negative and the neutral. Our Creator was well aware of these facts when he made us. He put on top of our bodies the governor – the head. Within the cranium are the important governing glands. It is through the use of cranial balance that one can balance these master glands and directly affect the others. The cranial bowl (head) is the superior positive pole of energy. Literally, we balance ourselves on our feet, also a most important area, able through zone therapy to affect the endocrines of our body. The feet are the negative pole of our energies.

We also have two other very important appendages, our hands, with their finer attachments. There are areas in our hands, acupressure or reflexology points, that can produce a beneficial effect on our endocrines. The hands are the neutral or neuter pole of energy.

The principle of polarity in the human body is the action of the finer energies in nature which work like atomic energy on radio waves. The radiant waves of this innate energy of life and warmth sweep over every living cell as an attraction and repulsion current, which is the prime mover in embryonic cellular life, long before it reaches the nervous system, which controls specific function and action.

This primary motive energy of life is a triune principle in operation, as male (or positive) and female (or negative) and a neutral pole as the child, as well as the origin of both poles in the beginning. So, the first is the last in the process of creation.

It is only since the discovery of the atom that we have been able to prove the actual presence of this function in every particle of matter, including the human body. The warmth of life, like the atomic heat, is transformed into chemical and mechanical action, guided by sparks of nerve energy to control its local and specific function. These finer forces in nature were seen as realities by the ancients. They are the key to the principles of health and its application in the body through manipulative polarisation, the lost art of healing.

The position of the embryo in the mother's womb is neutral. This is where the body is built and the energy pattern and design created here continue throughout life and develop the nervous system, the circulation, the glands and the muscular and skeletal structures. Our body is a microcosmos in a macrocosmos and is thus subject to all the physical, chemical and electrical laws that govern the universe.

Moon probes have shown that the Earth has an atmosphere and an ionosphere surrounding it, protecting us. These layers make up the fine electromagnetic energy fields that surround the planet. What happens in the ionosphere also takes place in our atmosphere. There is concern about what is happening to the ionosphere. The hydrogen bomb has ruptured our protective ionosphere, allowing ultraviolet and cosmic rays to come through which will injure our environment eventually.

Naturally, you will say, 'What has this to do with the electromagnetic field of our bodies?' Remember, your body is an extension of the earth – we have three finer magnetic fields:

1. the emotional electric energy field
2. the mental electrical magnetic field
3. the electrical magnetic field

Actually, the whole universe is a mass of electromagnetic light waves in gravitational movement. In other words, the universe, including the human form, is continually in a state of pulsating electromagnetic light waves as solid and liquid gases, but in reality these waves continually manifest as motion or vibration.

Disease means dis-ease, or lack of ease or harmony, lack of well-being. Emotion means a moving out of energy. These energy fields have to be normalised or balanced before the disease or symptom can be corrected. Disease is the result of disorganised electrical forces. Health is the result of the organisation of electrical forces – we must learn to organise these forces for healthful purposes.

If you refer to the diagram of the human body in the illustration provided, you will see that the plus (or positive) energy flows down the front of the right side, and negative up the back of the right side. In opposition, there is a negative (or minus) flow upwards on the front of the left side and a positive (or plus) flow downwards on the back of the left side. These flows of body energy are like two separate magnets, giving their respective polarities to the human body.

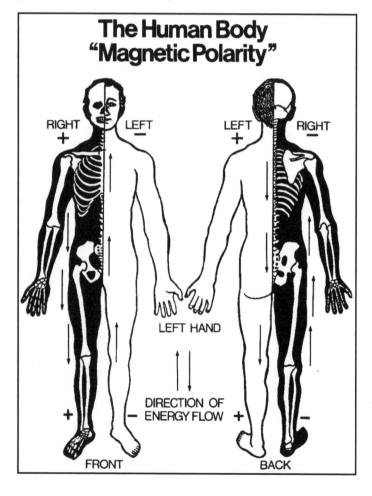

When Isaac Newton discovered the law of gravity, he was totally unaware that the very same law was a major contributor to the ills of man. Gravity starts pulling the human structure out of balance from the time it is an embryo until the day it goes to its grave. Much like the unbalanced wheel will cause a watch to stop or an unbalanced load will cause a ship to capsize, so an unbalanced body will cause innumerable ailments in the human being. George Ivan Carter, through years of study, inspiration and revelation, developed a simple, foolproof method of aligning the body structure and called it 'bone symmetry'. It is by this means that the human body may be brought into perfect balance and thus back to perfect health and normal operation. This scientific system has proven itself to be effective over a considerable number of years. Testimonies from thousands of people are evidence of the marvellous results it has had in helping human suffering. Carter came to the conclusion that in order to have harmony, peace of mind and health within the human body, perfect balance must be maintained in all the bones and joints.

Unfortunately, the stresses of life affect the nervous system, as well as the blood, and the muscles register this stress in tension. Very few of us pay any attention to our posture, but bad posture will produce a marked distortion and this will cause certain pressures which restrict the blood flow and ultimately the nervous function of the body. If people could only realise what misery and distress is caused to the human body by the mastoids and the neck being out of position! The neck sometimes becomes very stiff and sore and, if the middle bone of the neck gets out of alignment, it interferes with the teeth by cutting off the circulation and nerve energy, causing them to decay and the gums to become infected.

The first step in rebuilding health is to take the neck and shoulders into consideration. If the neck is crooked and the shoulders are out of alignment, it will change the position of the internal organs. The shoulder blades are responsible for the condition of the neck. If your right shoulder is lower and appears to be longer than the left, you will find the left shoulder blade to be an inch higher than the right. Upon examining the back of the shoulder, you may feel a large solid lump. The right shoulder blade has moved down and there is very little tension, if any, above the shoulder blade. The right shoulder blade will crowd the spine out of position to the left, or closer to the left shoulder blade. This causes the seventh cervical, or the large bone on the back of the neck, to move to the left. The cervical region, or bones of the neck, will pull to the right and cause the atlas, or top bone of the neck, to twist out of position. If you then closely examine the front of your neck, you will find that the right side of your neck seems to be a trifle larger and firmer. This is the starting point of trouble with your eyes, ears, nose and mouth, and migraine headaches. Your chest will become prominent, or very full on the left side, while on the right side, a depression will be noticed, which will interfere with your breathing. Such cases have been termed tuberculosis of the lungs. The reverse condition of the chest would indicate wheezing or asthma.

It is obvious to anyone who gives the matter attention that when one stands with the left shoulder lowered, the spine will move to a different position. Again, when the left shoulder is raised, the opposite one drops. This gives a quick and clear understanding of how the spine moves from one position to another and how rigid the ligaments will become inside the body under the higher shoulder. In this case the opposite side becomes so relaxed that it forces the internal organs of the body to move out of place and become congested.

If distortion is present, especially in the hand area, different parts of the body begin to move out of shape. A twist in the neck, or shoulders out of alignment, may interfere with the entire nervous system. Once a disturbance is aroused in the autonomous nervous system, the whole body produces some peculiar and dangerous symptoms which are normally (and wrongly) termed a disease.

I do not intend to give you details of the working of the nervous system – this knowledge can be gained from books in any library – but I hope your interest will be aroused and that you will go on to learn more about the workings of the body.

The complications produced by any distortion have far-reaching implications, due to an energy pull. The entire glandular or endocrine system can be affected. One must observe that the human frame always presents a clear picture of the individual who owns that frame. Blood pressures can be helped by means of observation and application of the 'bone symmetry' methods.

In a roundabout way, distortion of the human frame affects lymphatic drainage, which is even more important than blood flow. Very little has been written on this subject, so please bear with me while I go into more detail.

## THE LYMPHATIC SYSTEM

The lymphatic system is of great importance. The lymphatics are far more in number than the arteries and veins, and are connected with all parts of the internal organs. They are found in the skin of the body, face and scalp, and have a great influence on the thyroid gland. They carry the sense action to all parts of our body. The sense of taste – good or bad – is affected by the condition of the lymph. The lymph has a great influence on the movement of any part of the neck and hands. If it becomes thick and sluggish, it gradually slows up the action of the blood, as the gland supplies strength to the red blood. The more active the lymph becomes, the more quickly your body will move.

The lymphatic system consists of a complex network which collects the lymph from the various organs and tissues of the human body. It is a system of connecting vessels, which conduct the lymph from the different parts of the body to the large veins of the neck, connecting with the jugular vein and veins of less importance, where it is poured into the bloodstream. In the system of connecting vessels, there are many lymph glands or nodes; these little nodes or sacs, acting as filters and separating one substance from another, resemble buttons on a string and are placed apart at different distances.

We will start with the head and face, drawing an imaginary line from the throat, back to meet with the third cervical (the bone in the middle of the neck). We find these strings of lymphatic nodes coming out from the deeper tissues and travelling through the flesh on the face and head, beneath the skin. One branch travels up the jaw to the eye, while two other branches travel to the nose. Two important nodes lie between the ear and the cheekbone, in line from the ear to the point of the nose. From here, the glands (15 or 20 in number) travel up both sides of the head. The duty of these glands is to collect fats and waste materials and carry them into the deeper portions of the body. Just above the collarbone on either side of the neck we find a group of these little nodes, five or six on either side, extending down into the deeper part of the body, and branches extend down through the flesh and connect with the shoulders. You can feel little nodes in many parts of the body.

The next group is located in the back of the neck, travelling up inside the skull, forming a drainage system and continuing from there down to the extreme lower part of our body. The temperature of our body depends greatly on the action of these lymphatic nodes.

Next there is the lymphatic system of the neck, starting beneath the chin, travelling along the two main arteries down to the breastbone (sternum). There is a group of lymphatics, which again look like buttons on a string, descending from the collarbone to the solar plexus. A little string of lymph nodes extends from the spinal column, branching out to the various parts of the flesh and diaphragm.

Next we return to just below the collarbone, where we find a large knot with branches running in different directions, travelling down beneath the flesh and extending into the armpit. From there, many lymphatic veins travel down the arm on both sides, but the largest group inhabits the palm of the hand and the fingers. Here, by feeling, we can notice the relation between the lymphatic group and the conscious system, which carries the sense vibration of our body. All that is necessary for you to do to trace the lymphatics is to draw one finger of your right hand along the corresponding finger on the opposite hand and you get a marked sensation.

The next group of lymphatics extends from the shoulders and is seated deeper in the flesh, extending down the trunk of the body, with branches going to the breast area. The entire breast is one solid network of glands, with the exception of the nipple. This network of lymphatics has a great influence on the mammary glands in women.

In the lower part of the back (lumbar region) we find a large lymphatic gland, similar to an artery. At this point, the gland branches out and has many nodes – a dozen or so. Other little strings of nodes extend down into the lower part of the body to the fallopian tubes, ovarian glands, uterus, vagina and lower limbs. These glands collect the lymph from the lower extremities and carry it in the direction of the heart. There it makes connection with one of the main arteries and pours the lymph and chyle (milk-like substance) into the blood. The lymph is carried around the body by the circulation of the red blood until the blood passes through the kidneys, where toxic substances are extracted from the blood and then eliminated by the force of the urinary channels.

# THE SKULL AND FACIAL BONES

To take you a step further to understanding the far-reaching healing effect of bone symmetry, I will talk a little about the skull and facial bones.

The bones of the skull can move out of position for many reasons. First, consider the jawbone. If the left side of the skull is low, the right side is forced to rise out of position. This causes the teeth on the left side of the mouth to close much more firmly than on the right, and then we are inclined to chew our food on the left side of our mouth. By doing this, we take the pressure off the teeth on the right side, which will stop the nerve action and the circulation of the blood to both the upper and lower teeth on that side of the face. In many cases, this is the cause of ulcers of the teeth and toothache, or a condition called pyorrhoea may set in. If the lower jawbone is too low, then the cheekbone is also lower than it should be. This causes the sinus and facial bones to twist out of shape. By standing before the mirror and placing one finger of the right hand under the right cheekbone and one finger on the left hand under the left cheekbone, we can tell just how much the facial bones have moved out of position. Now this unnatural pressure of the facial bones will cause trouble in the antrums, also the adenoids, causing a stoppage in the sinuses.

In a close examination of the bones of your face, one eye may appear to be lower than the other. This is the case when the facial bones are out of position. If the bone of the forehead has moved down on the left side, the left eye will be lower. As the left side of the front part of the skull moves downward, it naturally causes the back of the skull on the same side to move upward. This will interfere with the position of the mastoid gland, bringing an unnatural pressure on the medulla and interfering with the sight and hearing, as it causes the mastoid bone to rise, corresponding with the back of the skull. This movement will prevent the head from being in a straight position upon the atlas (top bone of the spine), impinging the nerves of the spine and causing a lack of energy in the brain, eyes, ears, nose and throat. Thus, to a certain extent, the circulation is cut off to the different parts of the head and face.

People who are not sure of their step occasionally miss their step and fall, or their ankle will turn. Others stagger at times, or are afraid to go to high elevation, or to climb a ladder to unreasonable heights, or they look down from the top of high

TREATING BODY, MIND AND SOUL ~

buildings, exclaiming, 'Oh, this makes me dizzy.' The cause for all this interference is located in the brain directly under the temporal bone, which is just above the ear. If the left side of the forehead is low, it brings a pressure on this bone, crowding it in, in turn pressuring the brain. This same bone on the opposite side of the head will protrude, causing fullness on the right side of the head. All this brings pressure to bear on the centre of balance in the brain. This pressure not only causes the above troubles, but also unbalances the whole system – the thinking, the will and the action of the entire body.

If the skull is higher on one side than the other, it will cause a pressure on the brain, stopping the function of this portion of the brain and the nervous system that connects with some of the vital parts of the body. The skull moving out of position is often responsible for the appearance of lymphatic tumours in the scalp.

If the forehead is out of alignment, one side higher than the other, you will readily notice it in the bony structure above the eyes. If there is a depression in the skull, just behind the forehead, it will cause the neck to become stiff, the shoulders to move out of alignment, and much trouble to arise in the hands and wrists. On each side of the top of the skull, there is a direct connection between the underlying portion of the brain and the feet, especially the toes and metatarsal arches. If a defect appears in the back of the skull, we may have trouble with both eyes and ears. The misplaced bones will cause pressure on the brain, or the cells of the brain connected with different parts of our body. There is also an opening in the top of our skull through which we make spiritual contact with the rest of the universe.

Now, just consider the misplaced sections of the skull and the great influence and pressure they bring to bear on the nerves and circulation of the head and face, and on different sections of the brain. It may take a number of treatments to return the skull to a perfect condition and relieve the nerves and the circulation of the red blood.

## THE MASTOID GLANDS

The mastoid bones are located just behind the ears and continue back along the base of the skull (they are located between the temporal and occipital bones). Like the other divisions of the skull, they sometimes move out of position and cause considerable trouble with hearing. If the left side of the skull moves forward, it interferes with the hearing of the left ear, causing considerable trouble with dry wax. It's also possible to find the same disturbance on the right side of the skull and ear.

Ordinarily, we do not pay much attention to the mastoid bones, but when we take them into consideration, we find that they are of great importance, as inside them are air chambers similar to the sinuses in the front of the head. The interior of the lower part of the mastoid bones consists of small cells resembling those of a honeycomb. These cells contain marrow and hormones of different kinds which provide lubrication for the ear and eventually become a waxy substance. If there is a disturbance in the red blood cells, or a lack of circulation, the heat ratio in the mastoids and ears will decrease. The shell, or the outside, of the mastoid bones is almost as hard as ivory.

The mastoids play a large part in our hearing. The two mastoid bones are connected by tissue. This tissue extends forward, making a connection with the inner eardrum. The outer eardrums connect with the mastoid glands, which are directly behind them. These glands are not as noticeable in children as they are in older people. If there is an interference in the ears caused by the mastoid glands, it also interferes with our sight, taste and smell. If the skull is deformed or out of place, it will bring pressure to bear on the mastoid glands, interfering with the medulla and affecting the sense of taste and smell. The seat of sight is located in the back of the head near the mastoid bone. If there is an unnatural pressure on this bone, it will dim the sight of the eyes.

In many cases of eruption in the mastoid bone, a fever or inflammation appears. This causes a soreness of the bone behind the ear, causing enlargement of the mastoid and interfering with the tongue and throat. One gland from each mastoid extends down the throat and attaches to the collarbone. A feverish condition of the mastoids may result in many disorders, including throat trouble, causing large deposits of phlegm or mucus in the throat. Such conditions may be indicated by a very bad odour of the nostrils. There is another connection to the mastoids – a small acute gland travelling upwards, just behind the ear. It is sometimes referred to as an inferior duct and, in many cases, is surgically removed by an operation. However, the removal of this little gland may cause serious trouble in the brain, as blood poisoning can then develop in the mastoid. The position of the back of the skull has a great influence over the mastoid and glands.

## BONE SYMMETRY

George Ivan Carter had a rich knowledge of the human body. That knowledge was often so profound that it was inexplicable, but it was very ordinary in application. He expressed himself simply. One of the things he said was that every organ of the body will indicate its condition by a symptom. When there is trouble in the eyes, ears or throat, for example, you will find cold spots on the head, the back of the neck, the shoulders and arms, and right above the affected areas of the body. Each organ perspires, just like the brow, and if for any cause the perspiration is checked, a cold spot develops. If the liver is not working properly, there will be a cold spot over the liver, as the action of the sweat glands has stopped. As the perspiration leaves the body in other areas, there will be a peculiar odour indicating retarded action of the liver. At times, the odour of the body may be like that of the stomach, bowels or kidneys when passing a motion.

You can locate the cause of the trouble for yourself by passing the palms of the hands over the flesh. When you come to a cold spot, you will know that the organ beneath needs attention. If the gall bladder or gall duct are impaired, you will find a cold spot on the right side of the body, just at the bottom of the diaphragm, near the bottom of the ribs. Your spleen is also of great importance. You will find a cold spot, when the pancreas and the spleen are affected, on the opposite side of the body – the left side – just at the bottom of the ribs. Practitioners should put their right hand on the ribs when treating the pancreas and spleen.

If the cause of distress is the breathing or respiratory system, right at the end of the breastbone you will find the centre for the solar plexus, which when treated will take care of the breathing very quickly. The solar plexus is the greatest nerve centre of the body, from which groups of nerves extend to every organ. When you treat from this centre, you will immediately feel the warmth of the minerals passing into the body, into each and every organ.

Our thinking faculties are divided into three separate parts – objective, subjective and subconscious. Our thinking is transferred from the universal mind to the three divisions of our brain. Our thoughts, actions and deeds depend greatly upon the action of our conscious system upon our brain. If the organism of our body is not functioning properly, it interferes with the communications from the conscious system to our brain,

46

causing heavy, sluggish thinking. Torpid liver, gall bladder trouble, constipation and many ailments interfere with the consciousness and detract from the action of the brain. In this book we will see that many different bodily influences can and will interfere with our thinking.

Various parts of our body have a direct connection with the brain. A skull that is out of position may interfere with any natural talent we have. If the temples are out of position, it is very easily detected by moving your hands slowly over the skull – you will discover a groove or uneven surface. If the parietal bones bulge on either side, it will cause pressure on the nervous system of the entire body, causing a person to worry or fear. If the frontal bones are moved far enough out of position to cause pressure on the frontal part of the brain, it interferes with the intelligence. If the lower division of the skull in the back of the head (occipital) moves downward the slightest bit, it will cause pressure on the mastoid gland, and this will interfere with the hearing. The same condition may cause serious eye strain. If these pressures are brought to bear on different parts of the brain, it interferes with our thinking.

If we have an understanding of our thinking and hearing, we can use the mind to a greater extent. There is but one mind, the universal. It passes through the three divisions of our brain. If our brain is clear of bodily pressures and interference from the nervous system, we can translate the universal mind into thinking. Its vibrations pass through the front part of our head. Through this we may access some very valuable thoughts which could bring to us information that we have been seeking for years. Many things that previously seemed very confusing and hard to understand will be made plain to us through clear thinking. This demands uninhibited action of the brain.

In order to have a clear brain, we must have a body that is functioning properly, free from aches and pains, constipation and indigestion. Our lymphatic system must work properly, the flesh and skin must carry out their duties without interference, our conscious system must be free from depression, and our liver, gall bladder, pancreas and spleen must function properly. We must reconnect our body and our soul before we can think correctly, both physically and spiritually. We should be very careful when translating mindfulness into thought.

As Dr Allan often said, 'Man is immersed in a sea of energy forces that circulate about him and directly affect the balance of his health.' These forces are vital and without them we cannot exist or survive. The glands function as the governing gear of an engine and every time we heal it is an intelligent act, involving the use of forces we do not really understand. Hippocrates, the Father of Medicine, put it wonderfully when he said, 'Health is the expression of a harmonious balance between various components of man's nature, environment and ways of life. Nature is the physician of disease.' This particular doctrine is still vitally important today. One has to become body-wise and learn to listen to the body when problems surface. The last thing I want is for readers to become hypochondriacs or neurotics, but you should learn to listen to the body in quietness and then take appropriate action. We should think about what our body is doing, how we hold ourselves, how much we are in balance, and what has gone out of harmony. The body must be seen as a physical expression of a person's mind and soul, manifested in the thoughts. Biofeedback on the body is very important. I am often amazed, when positive action is taken on a long-standing problem, how quickly things can be adjusted. At the end of this part of the book, there are some case histories of people who have experienced great benefits following a minor adjustment, showing that the body actually wants to heal itself. It is very sad when people come to the stage that they disown their body and believe that they just have to live with their health problem.

Many forces affect us all the time and can put us out of balance. When the load is too much on one side of the body, such an imbalance very often leads to more serious problems. Almost on a daily basis, since I appeared on television and adjusted somebody's jaw, I have been consulted by people whose jaw has been put slightly out of position after visiting the dentist. The effect of this can be devastating, for the TM (trans-mandible) joint and hyoid bone may both be affected, and this can even make a difference to one's voice. I saw this clearly with a very famous singer who came to me for treatment when she noticed that her voice was not what it had been following a slight jaw dislocation. It only took seconds to put the jaw back into place and the result was tremendous. To this day, when I hear the singer's beautiful voice, I am happy about the difference that very small adjustment made.

I once heard a lecturer in Amsterdam say that we should simply sit down, breathe in deeply, feel the life force going through our body, feel every bit of the body, and then ask ourselves what doesn't feel right. The answer is always within: the body will tell us. Energy should flow freely, for it is essential for vitality and functioning well in everyday life. I saw this once with a priest who, for a number of years, had great problems celebrating mass. In the middle of it he would get stuck. A nagging pain around the sigmoid area was often the cause of his problem. With the use of a one-needle technique I learned from a Japanese professor, this priest, whose energy was slightly blocked, was cured and never had to suffer that dreadful experience during mass again.

Gravity is an energetic flow which keeps our balance stable. It affects us constantly, for instance when walking straight, standing straight and functioning smoothly. It is essential that even the smallest thing that affects our body's gravity be adjusted, for movement is the expression of everything we do.

Health is a dynamic equilibrium. Whenever there is an imbalance in the body, we have to look at the root cause in order to find out where an adjustment needs to be made. With all the tensions that life brings nowadays, I often find the body being attacked by negative forces. As well as a healthy diet and plenty of sleep, exercise is absolutely necessary. Even if you do not have time for anything more strenuous, you should always make time for walking, swimming and cycling. Of course, there are also wonderful, gentle forms of exercise like Rolfing, Alexander technique, feldenkrais, pilates, yoga and many others. It is also very important to carry out my famous Chinese breathing exercise technique which I shall explain in the final part of this book. Body knowledge is very important. As I have already said, avoid being a hypochondriac, but listen to what your body is trying to tell you.

Satisfying our basic needs requires movement and exercise. Hunger, thirst, shelter and reproduction all motivate us for survival. The physical body deteriorates without movement. The laws of nature compel us to be active, physically, mentally, emotionally and spiritually. None escape this universal drive. The energising fuel we need for our nutrition to do its work is oxygen. Without it, life ceases within minutes. Life (and death) occur on a cellular level; the chemical reactions which take place in individual cells depend upon oxygen for combustion.

Metabolism is the sum total of all the processes related to the building up (and tearing down) of the cells. Proper fuel, and oxygen, need to be circulated to reach all the billions of cells that make up the various glands, organs, blood and lymph. It is for this purpose that the circulatory system is called upon as a carrier of both fuel and oxygen. As air is breathed in, oxygen is separated and carried to the bloodstream, and carbon dioxide is exhaled along with vaporised water. As the oxygen moves in, carbon dioxide moves out. When oxygen is even mildly deficient, toxins accumulate in the blood and lymph, and will ultimately poison the cells.

For efficient circulation of the blood, nature has provided the heart with two pumps. One pushes the blood through the lungs (for oxygenation), the other circulates it to benefit the rest of the system. For this, it has help: with each expansion and contraction of the muscles, arteries, veins and capillaries produce their own pumping action; some veins have smaller valves of their own which are also activated through movement. At rest, all the blood in the circulatory system completes the circuit once in one minute, but it can do so as many as five times in one minute during exercise. Oxygenation, nutrients and waste removal all depend upon movement, circulation and activity. These processes allow cells to live and function, the brain to think and reason, the memory to be quick and alert, and the intricate functions of elimination of wastes to be consistent and regular.

Life is in the blood, according to the Good Book. To ensure adequate circulation, the body must be exercised. Expensive equipment is not needed, but group exercise is more fun and a greater incentive than boring press-ups. Walking is a great way to start – it may be practised in normal clothes or sports clothes. Walking reveals many things often missed when driving. It gives more time for thinking and planning, and more oxygen to the brain creates more creativity and imagination.

The lymph system is probably the most overlooked part of the circulatory system. To move the lymph, trampolining is excellent: start with 15 seconds every 15 minutes when you are at home. Gradually increase this to longer intervals. The short jumps at frequent intervals prevent too much toxic waste material being dumped into the blood at one time. It is when the body reaches zero gravity point and starts coming back down, by the force of gravity, that the lymph circulates effectively.

## MAN-MADE ENERGY

There is nothing in the universe except energy. How potentially harmful are some of the environmental man-made energies, and what is the responsibility of the government versus industry and free enterprise? Radio waves or frequencies have long been suspect when it comes to health, and there is literally no place on the entire earth where they can be escaped.

The Environmental Protection Agency (EPA) in America is now admitting its own concern (better late than never) and attempting to define 'limits of safety'. Paul Gailey, physicist with the EPA, and Charles Hall, an economist at Livermore Labs in California, have reported their findings. Gailey has measured radio waves and microwaves in 15 cities, using role models he developed to determine where the human body picks up such energies, like an antenna, most effectively. His conclusion: 99 per cent of the population is bombarded with one microwatt (or less) per square centimetre. What of the remaining 1 per cent of people? Gailey's measurements indicate that some people could be exposed to power densities thousands of times higher. His measurements were originally intended to determine if his models worked. In the process, he discovered not only that they did, but that the most likely source of high radio frequency fields affecting the public was related to FM towers. Gailey also showed that FM antennas emitted almost as much radiation straight down as they did out in the main beam. In addition, he stressed that FM stations – unlike TV – frequently use very short towers. Under the worst conditions (a high-powered station and a low-broadcast tower), it is possible to measure several milliwatts per square centimetre beneath an FM tower. And occasionally there may be a house there.

## RENEWING CELLS

Life is a constant renewal of cells, and I was quite taken by a lecture that a specialist gave in London some time ago. He was speaking on the monstrous subject of cancer. He emphasised how very important it was to renew cells. As I have said, up until the nineteenth century we knew very little about life. Today we know that life is a constant renewal of cell tissue and also how important it is that we not only exercise, but also have the right foods to eat and the right water to drink. This specialist said that the first thing he said when he woke up used to be 'Good morning, Elizabeth,' to his wife, but that now he says 'Good morning, cells that have kept me alive'!

It is interesting to note that the word 'cell' means 'to hide' or 'to conceal'. For more than two millennia, nature concealed her secret. Not until the development of the microscope were we able to observe cells and formulate theories on their structure and how they operate. Now we know just a little more of the secrets hidden within cellular fluids and the nucleus. We know that each of us begins life as a single cell, a fertilised ovum barely visible to the naked eye. By maturity, our cells total over several hundred trillion. Every 60 seconds, approximately three billion of these cells die, most on the surface of the skin. Miraculously, the majority of cells are instantly replaced by division of the remaining cells. Thus, the number of cells in the body remains fairly constant until old age or premature ageing begins.

Cytology and histology (the study of cells and tissues) have revealed some of the secrets of cell structure, content, biochemical individuality and nutritional dependency. The relationship between the nature of, and the presence or absence of, cells and various diseases, disorders and deformities is beginning to receive serious consideration.

A fairly healthy organism, given the right raw materials (minerals, trace minerals, trace elements, natural foods, complex carbohydrates, vitamins and enzymes from natural foods), supported by an efficient digestive capability, can – and will – sort, separate and combine (from the total available) what is needed to manufacture, on demand, replacement cells for the body while at the same time supplying energy for optimum activity.

Without question, certain vital elements for cell renewal are missing in refined, processed foods. There is some attempt to replace vitamin B and iron in refined cereals and flours. However, it is widely known that inorganic iron oxidises vitamin E and is poorly assimilated. What happens when even one essential raw material is missing has only recently been related to nutrition. One early recognition of the importance of the right nutrients came when it was realised that an adequate supply of vitamin B12 (folic acid) is needed in early pregnancy to avoid birth defects. It is now recommended that pregnant and nursing women ingest twice the recommended daily amount of folic acid for other adults. Some studies reveal that folic acid deficiency is widespread among both the 'well fed' and the underfed.

Cell renewal is so important and the responsibility is ours to make sure we receive the simple forms of energy which are so necessary for our state of well-being.

## MOVEMENT

Movement is synonymous with life: motion signifies the state of being. Thoughts and feelings are expressed through movement. The lips and tongue produce speech to interpret the pictures the mind conjures up, the hand transcribes the mind's visual image into words. Every movement, whether simple and automatic or studied and complex, is a sequence of skeletal contractions and relaxations woven by means of complex interplay between muscles and the nervous system. In addition, there must be flawless synchronisation and interaction of many muscles. For the simple act of picking up a book or dish from the table, arm muscles flexed at the elbow must relax to permit the forearm to extend. The shoulder muscles must stabilise, to support the weight of the outstretched arm as well as that of the object picked up. If the body must lean forward to reach the object, the muscles of the trunk and legs must compensate for the shift of the centre of gravity.

Every level of the intricate network of the nervous system contributes uniquely to motion. How the body produces voluntary movements is little understood and has eluded scientists for centuries. Nearly all movement involves both conscious and subconscious factors; the decision to pick up an object is willed, but most of the activity of muscle action required to complete the act takes place unconsciously. Edgar Adrian, the British physiologist, said, 'The mind orders a particular movement, but leaves its execution to the lower levels of the nervous system.'

The command to move a skeletal muscle originates in the brain and is transmitted over literally millions of neurons, the cells of the nervous system, to reach and activate the muscle. An axon, or a long fibre, extends from the cell body, along with one or more shorter extensions, dendrites. Neurons vary widely in size and in the arrangement of their axons and dendrites, and some are multipolar, meaning that they can transmit either motor or sensory nerve impulses. Rarer are the unipolar neurons, with one axon and one dendrite, found in the eye, nose and ear, for performing specialised sensory functions. Rarer still are the unipolar neurons in the spinal cord, the nerves of which have two projections that fuse together just beyond the cell body and then divide, by splitting apart, to form a distinct axon and dendrite.

Chemical substances called neurotransmitters provide the

means of communication between neurons, and between adjacent neurons lie synapses, small gaps about one-millionth of an inch wide. The axons of most neurons have tiny sacs at their ends which burst, spraying neurotransmitters around synapses. A single neuron may have thousands of synaptic contacts in its surface. Like computers and other electronic instruments, the human brain requires transmitters and semi-conductors for specialised tasks. Whole, natural, unrefined foods, provide the nutrients which are needed for this purpose.

Back in the '70s and '80s, Betty G. Morales from the Consumer Health Organisation in America taught me some simple truths which I have applied over years of practice in order to learn the body's real needs. Today, we live in a society where we sometimes ask ourselves, 'Have we reached the point of no return?' The challenge is marvellous – we can choose which foods to eat and what water to drink. We cannot, however, choose the air we breathe. We must keep putting pressure on governments to reduce pollution to the lowest levels possible, as its contribution to the tremendous increase of degenerative diseases is unquestionable. What are we going to do about it?

Pollution affects everyone all over the world, even the healthy Hunzakuts, whose natural lifestyle has become well known after a report by Dr Murray. The fact that they eat very little meat is due entirely to its scarcity. They have no choice in favouring a meatless diet! In Hunza, there is little grazing land to support domestic animals and no refrigeration in warm weather, so meat eating is limited chiefly to winter months. In their pursuit of meat, Hunzakuts often climb into the hills to drive down wild yaks. Their milk is about 50 per cent cream, so it makes excellent butter and cheese. When an animal is slaughtered, the carcass is hung from a tree and all the villagers partake while it lasts. Yak meat is mild and tastes like veal.

The favourite drink in Hunza is selenium-rich glacial water, wine or any alcohol being strictly forbidden since all Hunzakuts are Moslems. During the grape season, some of the fruit is juiced and left to ferment for the making of vinegar. If the juice is drawn before the fermentation is complete, it becomes a weak alcoholic beverage called Hunzapani. This is forbidden, but it is not unknown for some of the young men to indulge, a practice that is considered socially and morally disgraceful and shameful. The pure, natural water that they consume instead is actually a

Hobson's choice, for it is the only water available. It is laden with micro-minerals and trace elements, particularly silver. When water canals are changed in their directional flow, the remaining fine silt shines in the sunlight. It is the presence of silver, more than any other mineral nutrient, which the Hunzakuts claim protects them from heart disease.

It is marvellous that in the world today there is so much scientific knowledge at hand. But are we using it intelligently, and what are we doing with it? The body is wonderfully made, so haven't we got a responsibility to look after it?

I will look at a few case histories in this book, hopefully without boring you, of people I have treated and who have taken the right action to improve their health, and who have convinced me that our bodies are remarkable. Over the years I have seen a multitude of people with similar problems, but some cases relate very much to what I have written about in this section. People's lives can be ruined by seemingly small incidents that happen to them and ultimately cost them their lives, while others are unaware that one little adjustment can often restore their health completely.

A very sad case comes to my mind of a young family whose lives were ruined by completely unwarranted accidents. I often think about it. One Christmas a number of years ago I was with my family in our holiday home in a small place in the woods in Holland. Unexpectedly, the father knocked on my door, accompanied by his beautiful daughter. I had known the family for many years and he had been told that I was in the country. He asked if he could speak to me privately and, through tears, told me that his eldest daughter had become ill. The illness was quite mysterious and no proper diagnosis had been given. He told me he did not know what was wrong but, according to the symptoms, it appeared that she had muscular dystrophy. He felt he had come to the end of the road with the doctors' investigations. When I saw the girl I could clearly see signs of muscular dystrophy, but I could honestly say that in other ways she did not appear to have this illness. I carried out some blood tests on her and heavy metals showed up. In unusual cases, this can be due to dental amalgam, but I did not think that was the case with this particular girl. My detection job began. After some time, I found out that as children they used to play in a sandpit in their back garden, adjacent to a little shed which emitted smoke every day. After long investigations, we discovered that the man who worked there had been producing material for which he used heavy chemicals and also heavy metals. Following a further blood test, this poisonous material was detected in the girl's body. As a result of this my patient, now in her 20s, had become very ill, to the extent that slowly everything packed in. She became completely bedridden and was able to do very little. She could not use her arms and legs and, to cut a long story short, within a year's time could only communicate with her eyes, which was what kept her going. Unfortunately, an operation left her completely dependent on a life-support machine, which kept the poor girl alive for many years. There was very little pleasure left in her life, except to see her family. My best friend, Dr Hans Moolenburgh, managed to communicate with her in a very clever way and they wrote a book together. She could still hear, and listening to music was the only tiny bit of enjoyment in her life.

During this period, her equally good-looking sister came to see me with her husband. They had two lovely sons. She said that she did not feel well and asked if I could examine her. Knowing the family history, I became very suspicious and asked her to come with me to see a specialist in The Hague to find out if her illness was connected to that of her sister, remembering that she too had played in the sandpit behind their house. I prayed very hard that this would not be a similar case but, unfortunately, the blood test revealed the same problems. I was even more worried because she was pregnant. However, I managed to make her feel a bit better and got her through her nine months of pregnancy, and a beautiful child was born, which was a highlight in her life. Her sister, by now very ill, told her not to go through the same agony she had suffered in order to extend her life, only to end up barely existing on a life-support machine.

We had some very serious discussions about her future. I had to work really hard with her. She was so happy to have given birth to such a beautiful child, but this changed when she realised that she would not be long with us as her health deteriorated daily. A few months later, she died peacefully; there had been absolutely no hope for her.

I had a terribly emotional time with this family. They were the victims of today's society. I know that speeches on pesticides, herbicides, chemicals and pollution are often taken lightly, but it made me more determined to try to preserve the world as it was given to us, with everything in harmony. However, we have damaged nature to a great extent. It was so sad to see these poor children, who had played innocently, having their lives ruined by pollution. It is at such times that you realise just how precious life is, but also how quickly it can be taken away.

It is crucial that we keep the environment clean. What can society do to protect our children and preserve life? Does it become a matter of saving life at any cost? Over the years, on several occasions, I have gone through the ordeal of witnessing how terribly lives can be damaged. All too often, a great deal is said about how to help people die. In the world we live in today, with its rapid changes in values and standards, we see that ways which would previously have been effective are no longer adequate to solve the problems that arise. This scientific world has forgotten that we are all born in nature, we belong to nature, are part of nature and have to obey its laws.

In the past, every living being had its own space. More recently, over-population has become a problem. At first this was limited to certain regions and was often caused by wars and immigration, and temporarily relieved. The serious problem we face today is caused by the fact the world's population keeps increasing by an incredible amount each year. Despite this, as a result of natural disasters and the lack of food in the Third World, it is shocking how many people die of starvation every day. It is our responsibility to protect life and we have to work towards that goal, not only with normal healthy people, but also with the chronically ill.

Industrial procedures, with the immense technical and chemical processes involved, are causing more and more people to become ill. We listen to those who say how good it is that life expectancy has increased, but do we seriously consider the quality of life, rather than the quantity, when we see the terrific increase of degenerative diseases? Not only children, but adults too, are increasingly being harmed in more ways than one. In modern medicine, the side effects of concentrated chemical substances bring about new symptoms, which have to be eliminated by the introduction of other substances which, in turn, spark more problems. Combine this with an unnatural way of living and it is hardly surprising that our organism is incapable of processing and assimilating so many toxic substances.

In a way, if a patient becomes as ill as the girl I treated who was poisoned by heavy metals, it would be a blessing to die rather than face a life of suffering. When I looked at her, with tubes going into her nose and throat, and appliances to keep her breathing and fed, I often thought to myself, 'Is this life?' It was no life for her. The environment should therefore be preserved at all costs in order to protect one's health. This awful horror story is by no means unique. There are many similar cases throughout the world, where people are victims of today's science and research, where they are used as human guinea pigs and often become suffering victims. This is a problem that needs to be looked at seriously and we must realise the responsibility of medicine: doctors, surgeons and other health practitioners should see their job as healing and know that life, which is a gift from God, has to be handled very carefully and with responsibility. Action has to be taken for survival. If we consider the problem of starvation, which can even happen in normal circumstances or through illness, we will realise there is a huge job with only one solution – to try to keep over-population to a minimum, and to look seriously at medicine today and where we can improve it.

Every human body has free will and a right to its own destiny. The two sisters that I have talked about couldn't live by that principle. They were both committed to their Creator and had respect for life. I had some wonderful talks with them, which I will discuss in the third part of this book. Never in my life have I seen two young people who had death in their eyes, but apportioned no blame and were totally accepting of what had happened to them. They were so committed to what they believed, that it was not difficult to treat them.

I find it a daily struggle to help people improve their lives. When it comes to dietary management, for instance, it is probably easier to change people's mind on their religious or political beliefs, or on their husbands and wives, than it is to convince them to alter their eating habits.

Unfortunately, in our modern world compassion, dedication and human kindness have almost become foreign words. We need people who still have these principles and it is a joy when I come to treat those that do. It is right to have self-protection, but it is also very positive to commit oneself to making small, necessary adjustments. I often see, when I am able to change people's attitudes from being passive towards becoming more active, that step by step, they adapt more easily to life in the future.

This makes me think of a man who felt he was completely at the end of the road. One day a very impressive car arrived at my clinic in Holland. I looked through the window and saw a well-dressed gentleman, flanked by his chauffeur and another man, walking towards the reception. When it was finally his turn to see me, he told me that he was a government minister from another country and that he had a big problem. He had been told a week earlier that he had inoperable cancer and therefore needed help. He was advised to see me and find out if I could do anything for him. His story was actually quite interesting and I listened to him intently. He told me that about six months earlier he had gone to his dentist to have a tooth refilled and that some of the old filling had to be removed before it could be replaced by a new one. Following his appointment he returned home, quite happy. However, two days later, he felt something in his throat. He returned to the dentist, who had a look at it and told him not to worry because there was nothing wrong. After two weeks had passed, the man felt the problem was getting worse, so the dentist examined him again. He repeated that there was nothing wrong and prescribed a gargle. The gentleman returned home, quite satisfied. After a month had passed, though, he still felt there was something in his throat, so he went to his doctor, who had a look and said he could not see anything either, but that he would make an appointment for his patient to see an ear, nose and throat (ENT) specialist. Two weeks later, he visited the specialist who, knowing how important the gentleman was, had a very thorough look but, again, found nothing wrong. Another gargle was prescribed and the man returned home. He left things for another fortnight and then went back to the ENT specialist, who by this stage thought it might be a good idea if he saw a psychiatrist! So he went to a psychiatrist, who had a good chat with him and told him that there was nothing wrong with his mind and he was perfectly okay, but the best thing would be for him to have further investigations carried out. He then consulted a general surgeon, who examined him and found that there was a tumour in his throat which unfortunately was inoperable.

The story interested me and I carried out a test using one of the allergy-testing machines. The results indicated the presence of heavy metals. I then phoned a friend of mine, who is a consultant in one of the hospitals. I told him the story and he asked me to send this gentleman to see him so that he could carry out a scan. The conclusion was that my friend phoned me back to say that he had found something he suspected was a piece of dental amalgam, and this had triggered the cancerous process in my patient's throat. This was the result I had expected. My friend paid me a compliment by saying it was a very clever diagnosis, but asked what I was going to do about it. Fortunately, I had dealt with a slightly similar situation before and told him to leave the patient to me so that I could treat him. We were lucky to be able to isolate the amalgam that had originally caused all the problems and, to cut a long story short, after several treatments the gentleman got better and his tumour eventually disappeared. Through him and other government ministers, my wife and I were invited to one of the finest dinners I have ever been to by way of a thank you. It was a wonderful experience which we still speak about today.

I have seen many patients over the years due to the problem of dental amalgam. I remember the day that Victor Penzer (a dentist from the United States) and I went to Oxford University to plead with them on this controversial subject. Disappointingly, we got nowhere. Incredibly, though, when we visited an ex-chairman of the Dental Association, he told us that he would never put dental amalgam in his own wife's and children's teeth. Luckily, nowadays more is known on the subject and it is better understood. I have fought to combat this problem many times, and although I prefer to treat some patients by attacking any toxicity that might have been found in their blood, my advice still is to remove the dental amalgam and replace it with composite fillings. It would be wise to do so, especially if a dentist needs to carry out work on the offending teeth.

The reason I say this is dental mercury is a great deceiver. The Toxicology Center at the University of Tennessee is rated as the best in the USA. In their evaluation of the most toxic substances known to man, ranging downward from the least toxic, plutonium is listed as the most deadly: it is lethal to humans, even in the smallest amount known. On the scale, the level of toxicity of plutonium is measured at 1,900+. Mercury, used in silver dental fillings, measures on the same scale at 1,600, while nickel measures 600. (This data is taken from the book *How Safe are Silver Fillings?* by Betsy Russell Manning.) Ms Manning's book is well researched and referenced, with numerous case histories.

A typical one, reported by Hal Huggings, Colorado Springs, should be studied by every serious dentist, doctor and psychiatrist. It concerns a 17-year-old girl, once outgoing and popular, with high grades, who turned into a recluse and refused to be out of her mother's sight. Asked to describe her daughter's behaviour, the mother explained that she had suddenly reverted to child-like speaking and had an unnatural concern about death. Since the girl had already been seen by 50 practitioners, including cardiologists, allergists, osteopaths, gynaecologists, chiropractors, psychiatrists and psychologists, and had been hospitalised for tests, it cannot be said that her previous treatment had not been among the 'best' and most expensive.

Fortunately, a simple dental problem brought the girl into contact with a dentist knowledgeable in the myriad symptoms of mercury toxicity, who thoroughly checked her dental history, which included six small amalgam fillings. Many of her symptoms had been included in dental and medical papers and journals discussing mercury poisoning, but none had mentioned silver-mercury fillings as a potential or suspected source. The dentist began removing the girl's silver-mercury fillings at once and there was a steady, measurable improvement.

One problem, until more dentists are aware of it, is testing, which is not consistent in all patients. A general rule is to pay attention to the white blood cell count. Other tests that should be carried out include a blood chemistry profile, hair analysis for minerals, an electrocardiogram, body temperature, white cell morphological changes, urinary excretion of mercury, whole blood mercury levels, urinary vitamin C, specific gravity and pH, electrical current (amperage) generated in the oral cavity and changes. In some patients, changes appear in all areas, but not always in consistent or predictable ways.

After the removal of dental amalgam fillings and leaching out of the system, some patients exhibit toxic reactions which affect the peripheral nervous system, immune system and cardiovascular system. Mercury in the biological system appears to create or mimic many disorders in these three areas, and this should be taken into consideration.

I often have more success in treating patients after the removal of mercury amalgam, although I consider each case individually and do not advise every patient to have their amalgam fillings removed. It all depends on the individual case and also if any indications of allergies or poisoning show up in blood tests.

It is worthwhile thinking about the centre of gravity and gravity loss, discovered by Isaac Newton. If one little wheel in the watch is not right, the whole watch stops. Equally, if one little part of the body is not right, then the whole body stops. This reminds me of one day when I was practising in one of our ten very busy clinics and a young mother consulted me about her baby. She was a beautiful child, but while I was looking at her, before her mother could speak to me, she had a fit. I was quite alarmed and her mother told me that she sometimes had a fit every ten minutes. I asked her what had happened and about the medical help she had received. She told me that she had been to many doctors. The child had been on several epileptic drugs, but with very little success. I looked at this baby's beautiful face and, as a father and grandfather, my heart cried out. I wanted to help this lovely child. I asked the mother to tell me her child's history. It was quite sad, for she had been under severe pressure since the child was conceived. During her pregnancy, she was not only under family pressure, but her husband was shot not long before the baby was due. She had several complications and went into hospital and, unfortunately, when the baby was finally about to be born, a caesarean section had to be carried out. I looked at the baby, felt her skull and noticed that a little damage had been caused. I managed to carry out some cranial osteopathy and sorted out the problem with a minor adjustment.

Writing about that little baby, I am reminded of a young boy called Andrew. I saw him shortly after he was born. He looked such a lovely little chap, but I could see he had real problems. Cerebral palsy was diagnosed and while Andrew has been growing up, I have been treating him with several remedies, together with cranial osteopathy. While writing this book, I saw him coming up the stairs to see me with a tremendous smile on his face. He is six years old now and one of the brightest in his class. It is an absolute delight to see him, so happy and so well, and as normal as any other boy, going to school and determined that his problems will not hold him back. Often, a child's determination helps them greatly. I am happy to say that small adjustments can be a terrific help.

Sometimes it is very difficult to get through to a patient when they have lost the will to live. They get so disheartened with the unsuccessful treatments they have previously had and are unable to believe they have any future. Often, hard work and an awakening of their life force is needed, and it is important to encourage them not to give up hope.

I remember a lady who had been through tremendous traumas. She had almost given up and had tried to commit suicide three times. I told her she had a lot of work to do and must cooperate with me in every possible way. She was completely fed up and couldn't stand even thinking of this, until I managed to unlock a thought regarding food management. I had a little chat with her and, as she had been interested in nutrition, told her this was the first and very best friend she had to help her get better. I spoke to her about a low-stress diet, in which she was most interested. I talked about carbohydrates and proteins and the importance of balancing the two, and told her that a low-stress diet certainly did not entail eating a lot of protein. She wanted to know more and asked me a very unusual question: 'What do you think are the greatest enemies in life to health?' Off the cuff, I replied, 'I have seven: one, viruses; two, fungi; three, bacteria; four, allergies; five, parasites; six, poisons and seven, deficiencies through overeating.' This was the information she had been waiting for. How, she wanted to know, could one have deficiencies through overeating? I gave her a long explanation and told her that I had treated many of these deficiencies, and that it wasn't the quantity of food that was of the most importance, but the quality. As she was mainly concerned with food management, I said to her, 'Although there are seven enemies, I also have seven great friends for good health: one, food; two, water; three, exercise; four, sleep; five, light (sun); six, energy and seven, remedies.'

We had a chat about this and after I talked a bit more with her, I found out that she had a very nasty candida albicans, which is a yeast parasite, that had become very active. This can drain a patient, resulting in them not having an incentive to live, and even the black rings under her eyes alerted me that there was a problem. I could actually smell the candida, as I usually do, and carried out a simple test to confirm my diagnosis. I asked her if I could treat this for her, a suggestion she welcomed. Every time I see her now, she is willing to listen to what I have to say. This problem was easily solved – she altered her eating habits because she knew the value of dietary management and also took a few remedies that I prescribed. One of the simple remedies I used was *Devil's Claw* from Bioforce, plus a candida formula. I adjusted her diet by eliminating wine, yeast, cheese, mussels and chocolate. As I have mentioned earlier, usually persuading a patient to change their diet is difficult. However, this lady was willing to do what she could to help me treat her. Dietary adjustment plays a very important part in clearing the problem of candida.

Sometimes I ask myself, 'What are we doing today with medical science and where has the system gone wrong?' This question arose when I saw a policeman aged about 40. He came to see me and looked very well, but was in despair about life. He said he had a heart problem and could not work any more, and he was totally fed up. Even his domestic life had suffered from 12 years of worrying about his heart. I told him I would have a good look at his heart and after I went over his medical history and carried out some tests, I sent him to see a well-known cardiologist I was acquainted with. I mentioned to the cardiologist that I could not find anything wrong. He carried out all the necessary tests and also went into the gentleman's history. During the course of this, it was revealed that one evening when he was called out to a disturbance in a pub, he separated two men who were fighting and, in doing so, was hit on the head by one of them. Unfortunately, he was knocked unconscious. He had to be taken to hospital, where a young consultant checked him and incorrectly entered in his notes that he had had a cardiac arrest and that due to his heart problems he was no longer fit to work. This diagnosis stayed with him all those years. It is very difficult when erroneous statements are detailed in a patient's medical records, especially when this follows them around for life. Over the 45 years that I have been in practice, this has often happened and it is frequently the case that when a second opinion is sought and tests are repeated, some of these patients can be helped greatly. It is useful to have a complete review of one's health, especially when certain adjustments can quite easily be made to improve matters. This was a simple error, but it had caused the unfortunate policeman to be terribly unhappy for 12 years, reminding us that health is a very valuable inheritance.

Writing about these cases, it comes to my mind how incredible the working of the body is. One very busy Saturday afternoon, I received a phone call from the father of a girl who was in hospital, whom he said was dying. He begged me to see his daughter as this was her only wish before she convinced herself she was going to die. The father, mother and girl arrived at my busy practice. When she walked in I could see that, like the load on a ship going to one side, she was completely out of balance and something mechanical was wrong. I listened to her telling me that she suddenly felt unwell and could not eat, and had undergone all the various tests in the hospital but nobody could find out what was wrong with her. Although she could not eat, she had a pain around the end of the gullet. The energy chakras around that area are very forceful and this 17-year-old girl, because of the problems she had suffered, had it in her mind that she was dying, due to her reduced life force. She had consulted various specialists: some thought she had anorexia nervosa, others thought it was a digestive problem, but none of them could get to the root of her problem.

Her mother said that most of the medical people she had consulted thought it was all in her mind, but I could see clearly by looking at her that there was a mechanical problem. I made an osteopathic adjustment slightly under the gullet, after which she said she felt some relief. I also carried out bone symmetry and further adjustments, and prescribed *Centaurium* from Bioforce, which is an excellent remedy to aid digestive absorption and helps increase the appetite. I also gave her a tonic and some vitamins. Within two days, this girl was walking straight instead of being bent towards the right side. The comments from the hospital she had been attending were quite revealing. After a few days, the specialist came to her bed with a group of students. Fortunately her father was present. The specialist told his students that this girl was a typical placebo patient who really had nothing wrong with her, but had been to an alternative practitioner in whom she put her faith and, because of the placebo effect, had suddenly got better. Her father interrupted and said, 'If that is the case, why didn't you cure her, if that was the answer?' He continued by telling the specialist that he could clearly see mechanically what I had done to his daughter. The body is very well constructed, but every bit, every muscle and every bone, should be in the right place, otherwise disharmony can lead to big problems, as was the case with this young girl.

I saw that very clearly with a boy who was more seriously ill. He came to consult me with his mother, who was in great despair as he often fainted and became absent-minded. She had told her son to go to the doctor, which he did not want to do, but he had agreed to come and see me. When I carried out a simple test on him, I could see that things were not right. I told him to see his doctor immediately and actually phoned the doctor myself, because in my iridology test and personal observations, I could see that something was very wrong. In fact, he had a brain tumour. Fortunately an operation was possible, from which he recovered quickly, and his balance then returned to normal. He now enjoys a very happy and healthy life. Luckily for him, he came to see me at just the right time.

I am trying to convey in this part of the book how easily little adjustments can lead to big improvements. This reminds me of a minister's wife who came to see me after being diagnosed with muscular dystrophy. This is a very serious disease which can often lead to early death. Strangely enough, I did not think that she had the condition. Very little can be done about muscular dystrophy, but some people have reacted well to dietary management and a careful balance of amino acids. It took me a long time to find out this lady's medical history, so I asked her to come back in the evening (which I usually do if I want to set aside more time) and went over her whole history from birth. This can sometimes take between one and two hours. In this case, it took a long time. I was mystified but, during the last five minutes of gathering the facts together, the answer came to me. As I have often said already, you have to look, listen and feel. I realised that the lady had a spot of psoriasis around the second and third cervical vertebrae. She told me that it never cleared up and, for 17 years, she'd had to rub a special ointment onto that spot to keep it under control. I knew the ointment was a strong substance and, after sending her for tests, discovered that it had destroyed the nerve tissue right on the third cervical vertebrae, which controls the sympathetic nervous system. Initially, the treatment for the psoriasis appeared to be perfectly safe, simply involving the application of a little ointment on the psoriasis, but, day after day for all those years, it had caused damage to the extent that the lady walked like a cripple. You should check with practitioners, doctors and consultants to find out the side effects when using treatments over a long period and these should be well monitored.

This reminds me of the loss of one of my dearest friends. We had known each other since we were very young and even after we both got married, we still remained friends and travelled together many times. We often visited one another and as she was a doctor in the place I had a clinic, we would talk on our journeys about medicine, so I knew that she had quite a lot of health problems and was slightly asthmatic. We were planning to get together one evening for a little birthday party and a few hours before the party was due to start, she jumped on her bike to get some extra things from the local baker. A car knocked into her bike, causing her to go over the handlebars and land in the street, where she passed out. She was taken to hospital, where they diagnosed nothing more than slight concussion. However, she deteriorated rapidly. By the following day, she could hardly breathe. Her husband, who was a very well-known doctor, started to become extremely concerned and spoke to the consultant to see what he could do. He had been asking to see his wife, as she was very ill, but they would not allow it. This was such a pity, because I knew that she had problems with her spine and told him that an X-ray should really have been carried out. Unfortunately, she died, at the age of 38, leaving four children behind. The post-mortem revealed that as a result of her fall, the unfortunate young lady's ninth dorsal was very badly damaged and she had so much pressure on her lungs that they basically gave up. It was a huge mistake on the part of the hospital that they missed this and resulted in a totally unnecessary death. I keep stressing how important it is to look at a problem from every angle, especially when an accident like this occurs, so that nothing is overlooked and tragedies may be prevented.

We have to keep our eyes wide open. This reminds me of how wonderful life can turn out for people who have not only lost their vision in life, but also their sight. Recently there was a story in the newspapers about a father with a young baby. He had been blind but came to me for treatment and, when the child was six months old, for the first time in his life he was actually able to see his baby. When he consulted me he talked about his tremendous happiness at the possibility of getting his sight back and was quite euphoric about it. When I managed to calm him down, I explained that macular degeneration is not an easy disorder to treat. Fortunately, through acupuncture and various remedies I prescribed, some of his sight returned. I have monitored him for a number of years now and, luckily, he has retained a lot of his vision. It is astonishing to see the results that can be achieved with the new development of bilberry products, combined with herbal remedies and good dietary management.

In my book, *The Five Senses*, I said, 'If you lose one of your senses, you lose the sense of living and therefore the ways that this can be restored, and even when losing one sense, it is always important to investigate this and to adapt one's system.' This brings another patient to my mind, whom I saw today before writing this part of the book. He is a wonderful gentleman who has been a farmer for many years. A few months ago he consulted me and told me that he had been struggling with his sheep. He said, 'It is usually the black ones that are rough and cause trouble.' One particular sheep had been obnoxious and thrown him off his feet, and his knee was so badly damaged that a consultant had told him it was beyond repair. He could hardly walk up the stairs in my clinic. I recommended a remedy I often use, called *Joint Mobility Factors*. This wonderful remedy comes from America and helps when there is cartilage or tissue damage. The gentleman was very willing to follow my advice. I also gave him some acupuncture to help with the problem. I saw an expression of total happiness when I met him today, as he told me that he could climb the stairs quite easily. He had done everything possible, even the things I had asked him to do at home, in order to get some mobility back. It is never too late to seek help and it is important to follow any advice that is given. It is essential to find harmony when the enemies in our environment try to throw the body out of balance by causing problems.

A lady once went to an important meeting in London. She was quite upset about certain things that took place at this meeting and suddenly began to feel unwell. She fainted and was taken to hospital. They checked her over and over again and, after a little while, came to the conclusion that she might have had a viral attack. She was very dizzy. However, a very strange situation arose. When she fainted she had fallen on her back, not her chest, but her breasts suddenly became almost black, as if she had internal bleeding. This was checked for and nothing was found. The diagnosis was still that she had a virus. Her periods became very erratic and when I saw her, I felt that this virus might have caused a hormonal imbalance, which turned out to be the case. She was completely out of balance and became very nervous. As I have often said, if the plugs are in the wrong sockets, the system goes haywire. The train that leaves the station will only reach its destination if every plug is in the right socket in the signal box. If the plug is in the wrong socket, it might go off the rails and disaster can be expected. In the human body it is very important to get the basics right and try to readjust imbalances with the help of remedies like *Female Balance, Female Essence* or *Menosan*, to keep the hormonal system in tune, as I described more explicitly in my book, *Menopause*.

We often use the expression 'to go back to basics' and that is often necessary, a fact that was brought home to me the other night when I attended a very important music festival. I enjoyed listening to the different professional musicians, many of whom won prizes. Then, when a young boy of 11 performed a wonderful piece on the violin, in my mind I felt I played every note myself. The judge was right in saying the music was perfect – every single thing that the boy was supposed to do, he did perfectly. What was most amazing was that he played the entire piece from memory and did not need the help of music sheets. He then had to play a piece by Mendelssohn on the piano. It was an extremely difficult piece because of its very high and low notes and I felt nervous that he would make a mistake. The audience listened to this little boy, almost holding their breath, and when he was finished there was very loud applause. After he had completed his part, he was awarded a most important trophy for being the best in the festival. As this boy was, in fact, my grandson (the son of my eldest daughter), I was in a position to ask him a question. It was his answer that made me think. I said to him, 'Michael, how did you manage that? I was so worried that you would get stuck but you did it all so perfectly.' He looked at me and quite naturally said, 'Dumpy, you just have to get the basics right.' Isn't that true of life? Whether an illness is physical, mental or emotional, look at the basics and make sure they are right, adhere positively to what we should do and obey the rules of nature to get ourselves back in order.

It is sometimes necessary to concentrate the mind to get better and not accept illness, but do everything we can to help. In the second part of this book, we will study the mind and see how strong it really is. We have three bodies (physical, mental and emotional), all of which should be in harmony. We need to look at the body, not as one, but as three, to discover exactly how much these three bodies depend on each other to get the basics right. It pays dividends to invest in one's health. This can be seen clearly with arthritis, a condition that can be truly devastating.

## ARTHRITIS
Some time ago I did a seven-year study on arthritis in Holland

with a group of rheumatologists, working with a Romanian professor. He listened to me when I emphasised that so often with arthritis, emotional problems play a part. It is frequently said that crippling rheumatoid arthritis has nothing to do with the mind or the spirit. I saw this clearly and studied the condition with the professor very closely. I told him that I often found that the causes of arthritis, attacking bones and muscles, are not always inflammation, infection, allergy or heredity, but that often a few causative factors play a part:

1. chronic resentment
2. unhappy marriage
3. sex problems
4. career disappointments
5. daily frustrations with which the subconscious mind continually does battle
6. worries
7. fear in all its aspects

The list could go on and on. On this project, we worked together to make the evidence clear, backing up complementary medicine in its approach to body, mind and soul, and made some important observations. Many consultants, doctors and practitioners lose sight of the fact that each patient is an individual. Therefore, to achieve any measure of success, regardless of what modality be employed, one must individualise – *treat the patient and not the disease.*

Arthritis is a common label attached to all who suffer from this insidious complaint. What is overlooked, however, is the fact that the label merely describes a well-known set of symptoms. The primary causes of these textbook symptoms are also well known and can be divided and subdivided into many categories. It is futile to say that this or that is the cause of arthritis: many causes could be the culprit. The problem that confronts the practitioner when the patient presents themselves is, which?

Our modalities are determined by our diagnosis and our clinical experience. To prescribe infrared, radiant heat, diathermy, massage, manipulation, acupuncture, homoeopathy etc. in a vain hope of eradicating symptoms, without first recognising the primary cause, is nothing short of quackery. These shortcut methods may afford relief, but that is all. What then is the answer? It is found within the patient – individualisation.

No two arthritic patients are alike, even though the symptoms may be similar in their presentation and severity. Mr Jones's father died of cirrhosis of the liver, like his father before him. Mr Jones is a hard man and not easy to live with, expressing frequent outbursts of temper. Mr Brown, after 40 years' faithful service and loyalty to his firm, is passed over for a younger man. Mrs Smith, due to a womb malformation, lost her firstborn 20 years previously and still suffers from suppressed grief. Mrs Green's ancestors possessed an arthritic tendency, skipping a generation here and there, but forever lurking within the shadows ready to assert itself. And so we can go on individualising.

Emotional conflict, suppressed grief, hereditary disposition – all are contributory factors, producing in their train the well-known symptoms we choose to label 'arthritis'.

There is no panacea for arthritis, no easy road to success via man-made treatments, orthodox or unorthodox. This cannot be denied. Yet we may perceive a ray of hope through this gloom, if we fall back upon natural therapeutic philosophies, gleaned from Mother Nature herself.

Having discovered the primary cause from our patient and totally ignoring the symptoms which we know so well, how do we proceed? Arthritis, like every other disease, obeys a natural law, the transgression of which by the host immediately puts into operation certain processes, chemically and anatomically. These processes are determined and controlled simply by the impetus given to them by the measure of transgression, either physically or psychically. These proceed in the following manner: calcium enters into solution in an acid medium and is precipitated and deposited in an alkaline medium. This simple but profound statement provides the key to unlock the mystery of arthritis.

Medical literature tells us that the entire physiological range of reaction of the extracellular fluid lies on the alkaline side of neutrality. The blood represents one-quarter of the extracellular fluid. Its reaction is weakly alkaline. With an alkalinity increased above its normal weakly alkaline reaction, calcium is precipitated and deposited into the tissues and bursae.

Excess alkalinity (caused by a protein intake that is too high, visceral emotion, tension, environmental or hereditary factors) will promptly produce the precipitation of soluble calcium in the bloodstream throughout the organism, mainly in the bursae, throughout the life of the host. To reverse the process of solubility, we must employ a secondary agent. This agent is potassium. Just as chlorine (salt) disperses natural iodine in the body, so potassium disperses calcium. Honey, grapes, apples, cider and cider vinegar are a few items of potassium origin and can be employed advantageously, the latter in the form of fomentations to the joints.

### Arthritis and Fascia

An understanding of fascial relationships will give an insight to patients suffering with colitis, rheumatism, arthritis and other comparable complaints. I will delve a bit deeper into arthritic conditions here, as these have a tremendous influence on the bones and muscles and are affected by the three bodies: mental, physical and emotional. We see so many problems with arthritis and rheumatism nowadays. For this reason, I have written at length on the subject.

First, let us consider vitamin elements (all B complex vitamins) which affect the fascias:

> Thiamine: process of metabolism to the pyruvic acid stage
> Riboflavin: continues process, then lactic acid stage into $CO_2$ and $H_2O$
> Niacin: reactivates activity of thiamine and riboflavin

If the vitamin elements are not present in the proper form and amount in the proper place, the patient has a chemical situation whereby the fascias and muscles are overloaded with pyruvic and lactic acid. The results set up an irritation of the fibrous tissue with inflammatory reaction and swelling.

Now, where does the body acquire its vitamin B complex? It is known that the small intestine, with the secretions and bacteria present there, functions as a factory. The result of the manufacturing, by proteolytic enzymes, digestive ferments, bacterial activity and chemical synthesis is the production of the elements needed by the body. This is a process of interchangeability of energy and matter.

If the fuel put into the intestinal tract contains vitamin B complex, the work is easier, but normally the process can be completed anyway. 'Normally' means having an abundance of the necessary ingredients to do the job, so that the end product of the manufacturing process is suitable for the work to be done.

### The Importance of Fascia

The following is intended to show the tremendous importance fascia plays in the life of the individual. From the cranial base, the fascia is suspended and continues in its lateral borders the carotid sheath or canal within which are the internal jugular vein, the carotid artery and the vagus nerve. This nerve is vitally important in the influencing of the activities of the stomach, small intestine, pancreas, liver etc. Anteriorly, the fascia attaches above and below to the hyoid bone, distally it continues to the posterior surface of the manubrium and at the manubrium sternal body junction, so it is in close relation to the clavicular and first and second ribs articulated with the sternum. Posteriorly, the fascial border goes distally and attaches or blends with the anterior spinal ligament at the level of the second thoracic vertebrae. Above, it is suspended from the basi-occiput. This tells us that sphenoid–basilar relationships and second dorsal lesions are in reciprocation, and the sympathetic nerves can be profoundly affected by alterations in their environment resulting from fascial stresses in this area. However, it is good to remember that every part of the body is maintained in a state of reciprocal tension by means of the fascia and the automatic shifting of the fulcra therein.

If the pancreatic duct, the duodenum, the bile duct and ampulla of Vater are disturbed in their normal relation, then it is axiomatic that their function is interfered with in such a way that the end product is not adequate to do its required job. That is when a patient presents symptoms.

## EFFECTS OF ALL FASCIA

From the posterior manubrial area, the fascia attaches to the pericardium and with a free retrosternal space it is attached to the xiphoid-sternal body area, the pericardium (anterior surface, distal posterior) and the diaphragm. Beneath the diaphragm is the attachment of the psoas sheath of fascia that extends all the way to the lesser trochanter of the femur and is also related by fascial connections to the second sacral segment and the pelvic fascial diaphragm.

A deviation in any one or more of the areas would automatically affect all the fascia and thereby produce a disturbance manifested somewhere by the patient in a variety of ways. This happens because the body is a complete functioning unit and gives us an insight into why and how patients with colitis, rheumatism, arthritis or any one or more of a large number of variable complaints can start to have problems.

The fulcrum of the fascia of the body may be considered to be secondarily at the attachment of the second dorsal and at the posterior manubrium and primarily at the Sutherland fulcrum (the sacrum).

The structure of the human body, more specifically the anterior convergence feature of certain structures, is an asset in permitting the above to occur as a part of the body physiology.

It is true that in applying the principles, one can put a part of the mechanism into a prelative or absolute conformance to the lesion present anywhere in the body and the entire mechanism will conform to the specific lesion pattern, and then the release brought about by the mechanism factor via the fascia. Points in the primary mechanism could be contacted cranially or sacrally, and secondarily sternally, acetabulary, at the second dorsal or wherever anterior convergence is a factor. If you can restore a healthy interchange of the interstitial fluids in the fascias of arthritics over a period of weeks and months, you can heal the problem.

## ARTHRITIS AND RHEUMATOID CONDITIONS

The literature on arthritis, although it is abundant, is very unsatisfactory. Most writers seem to have no concept of its real cause and, therefore, can suggest no sensible treatment. Despite all that has been written on the subject of arthritis, it is still an enigma as regards effective treatment. Before I attempt to describe techniques for the treatment of rheumatoid conditions, I think it is vitally important that we first review some background relative to the conditions that create the problem, then preliminary measures to be instituted in order to make the body receptive to osteopathic manipulative change and, finally, the specific general and local treatment.

An unfortunate pessimism about the possibility of a cure for unhappy sufferers seems to have arisen. The general consensus is that they have no choice but to live with their affliction the best they can. Modern medicine has openly stated, 'We do not know what arthritis is, therefore we have no effective cure for it.' Arthritis, in all its forms, is basically a nutritional or metabolic aberration. It is the result of the inability of the body to make available or to utilise the necessary biochemical elements ingested by it. This, then, results in an accumulation of metabolic wastes which settle in various tissues, especially the joints, giving rise to pain, stiffness, swelling and deformity. The chemical aberration varies in different individuals. This is the difficult part: finding chemical tests and diagnostic aids which will determine the patient's individual disturbance. Treatment should then be directed at correcting the diagnosed aberration.

The question is asked, 'How does the arthritic's metabolism become imbalanced in the first place?' There are three main factors:

1. an inherited abnormal chemistry or metabolism from the parents
2. the patient has had 'self-limiting' diseases of childhood (measles, mumps, chickenpox, etc.). Even though recovery is made, the effect remains, and this exerts an influence on their health for the rest of the patient's life
3. injuries from falls and accidents, especially to body joints

I have long been satisfied that rheumatic suffering comes entirely from the chemical action of poisonous fluids that should have been normally excreted from the system. I think it is an effect which is the result of impure compounds carried to, and deposited in, the vicinity of the joints in any part of the body.

When any part of the body receives a jolt as the result of a fall, a mental or physical shock or a wound, many kinds of abnormal compounds and fluids are produced, confused and brought together, and circulate in the system. If these abnormal fluids are not returned on time, but are deposited in the membranes, then congestion, fermentation or decomposition of the impure chemical compound follows.

When venous blood has been obstructed and retained in the region of the spinal cord and the cerebellum by impingement, or by muscle contractures operating to hold the upper cervical bones out from their normal positions, we have a condition that will result in rheumatism. Preventing the return of blood from above the articulation of the atlas with the occiput until stagnation sets up in the venous blood will result in heat and inflammation. Constriction and stoppage of blood at this area long enough will form poisonous compounds that take the place of healthy nerve fluid which should come from the brain. This poisonous fluid, taken up by the pneumogastric and cardiac nerves, is soon distributed to the entire body and this delivery of impure fluids results in a stagnation in the heart, liver, kidneys and the entire excretory system. Here the mystery of rheumatism disappears. This applies to both acute and chronic rheumatism. Open the gates and let the bondman go free. I have worked according to this theory and the results have been good.

The preliminary measures to be instituted in order to make the body receptive to change should follow a basic plan of treatment. Outlined, it would be like this:

### Stage 1: History
*Physical Stress*
a. exposure
b. loss or gain of weight
c. disturbed gastrointestinal and glandular function
d. fatigue
e. poor nutrition
f. acute and chronic infections (especially self-limiting)

*Mental Stress*
a. domestic and family problems
b. business and financial worries

### Stage 2: Physical Examination
a. laboratory
b. X-ray: both should be sufficient to get a complete picture of the patient

### The Treatment Programme
1. Patient orientation and understanding of the problem. The first and most important step in the treatment of the arthritic after examination is to obtain the cooperation of the patient by a detailed explanation of the proposed treatment programme.

There are two approaches to the treatment of the arthritic patient. This is contingent on the nature of the patient. Successful treatment requires that the doctor either knows the traits of the patient or talks frankly with them and determines if they are willing and/or capable of carrying out the treatment regime which is directed at reversing the degenerative process and attempting to aid nature in the reconstruction process.

2. If the patient possesses the intelligence, understanding and willingness to cooperate, then the total programme may be instituted.

3. If the patient is only interested in relief of discomfort, and lacks the intelligence to realise that this is merely the result of the condition and not the cause, then the treatment would be to palliate with the various drugs that are now available for that purpose, and try to interest the patient in as much of the reconstruction programme as you can. However, there are many people who are just not interested and you would waste your time trying to educate them.

4. Medication – to relieve pain and discomfort. Despite the many new drugs available for the relief of arthritic discomfort, aspirin is still the drug of choice. However, when aspirin or the salicylate-containing compounds are used, it is advisable to add ascorbic acid, as this helps prevent the excessive destruction of vitamin C by the salicylates.

5. Removal of any foci of infection, although this does not hold the important position it once did. Nevertheless, it cannot be overlooked.

6. Eliminate excessive weight.

7. Counteract anaemia.

8. Adequate rest and sunshine.

9. Exercise – this should be tailored to the individual case and requires specific instruction.

10. Bowel management – this is important, as all arthritics have trouble in this department: a. correct existing constipation and b. overcome digestive disorders.

11. Strengthen nervous system.

12. Normalise circulation of fluid systems.

13. See that, in particular, liver, skin and kidneys function normally. This phase of treatment and the preceding three play a very important part in techniques for the elimination of metabolic wastes and toxins, which are absolutely necessary before maximum results can be expected from manipulative osteopathic treatment.

14. Put patient on a nutritional programme, designed for the individual, which will provide adequate nutrition from easily digestible foods with a minimum of metabolic wastes. Because of the difficulty in obtaining high-quality foods (foods that are grown on fertile soil, which would contain the necessary minerals for cellular metabolism, and which are free of poisonous sprays and poisonous chemicals added to prevent spoilage in the food) it is desirable to supplement the diet with preparations containing minerals, vitamins, amino acids, enzymes and lipids. By thus adding to the regular diet, you ensure the body has an adequate supply of these important nutritional elements. Vitamins A and C are especially important to the integrity of the intercellular cement substance in connective tissue. Specific foods to be avoided in arthritic conditions are: coffee, all kinds of white flour products (white bread, cakes, rolls, muffins, buns, doughnuts, biscuits) and concentrated sugars (such as sweets, icing, ice cream and soft drinks). All sugars should be used sparingly. Other things that should be avoided are: mustard, pepper, sauces, ketchup, vinegar, excessive salt, spices and any pickled, preserved, smoked or otherwise highly processed foods. The patient should be given a list of foods they *can* eat. It is not enough to say what they *cannot* eat.


Manipulative management should be divided into General and Local:

### General
Must be atraumatic in nature and directed at:
1. Stimulating the general physiological functioning of the liver, kidneys, skin and glandular system, especially the parathyroid glands.

2. Establishing normal body fluid balance by stimulating arterial blood flow to all tissues, increasing venous drainage, aiding lymphatic drainage and balancing cerebrospinal fluid fluctuation.
   By thus effecting a more normal functioning of the vital body forces, we will promote the ability of the body to utilise the ingested elements from a carefully selected nutritional programme. Before the desired results can be expected from osteopathic manipulative treatment, it is necessary to eliminate

the toxic end products or metabolic wastes that have accumulated in the tissues, especially the joints, causing swelling, stiffness, restricted motion and pain. This is done by fasting, sweating, colonic irrigation and enemas. The large bowel is the source of much toxic absorption. Exercise, fresh air and sunshine will increase the oxidation of body tissue. Eliminate all but simple, nutritious substances from the diet.

It must be remembered that the manipulative treatment of the arthritic is strictly individualised to the specific patient, and the specific areas and degree of involvement present. It is therefore necessary that we talk in rather general terms about the manipulative therapy.

When possible, I like to treat the arthritic on my table. I would use a ten-degree slant, with the head lower than the feet. The purpose of this is to reverse the force of gravity and permit the body fluids to change position, thus encouraging drainage of blood and lymph by a simple change in posture. With the patient in this position, I give the general treatment. I place the chief emphasis on stimulating the liver and spinal areas controlling the parathyroid glands.

Great emphasis is also placed on treating the sub-occipital area:

1. Stimulate liver activity by placing one hand on ribcage under the liver and the opposite hand on ribcage above. Gently lift with the underneath hand and, while lifting, compress or approximate with the above hand and introduce a slight vibrating movement into this procedure.

2. Attempt to normalise the spine between cervical seven and dorsal four. This is the area of influence on the parathyroid glands.

3. Gently relax and establish motion (not necessarily bony corrective motion) in the sub-occipital area. The reason for this is to try and improve the exchange of fluids from within the cranium to the tissues of the spine. This 'nerve fluid' holds an important position in the mechanism of maintaining health or producing disease. I visualise this fluid as cerebrospinal and health is dependent upon it reaching the tissues of the body, as nature intended it. Since most people do not fully understand the mechanism of its transportation, they consequently find it

hard to understand how this could have anything to do with the treatment of arthritis.

### Local Treatment to Joints

1. Gentle traction and attempting to put the joint through its normal range of motion by use of functional technique.

2. Heat and various physical modalities may be used, such as ultrasound, hydrotherapy, infrared rays and hot packs.

3. The purpose again in local treatment is to get an exchange of fluids directed at normalising blood, lymph and cerebrospinal fluid.

### Summary

1. Arthritis and associated rheumatoid conditions are basically metabolic disturbances caused by the inability of the body to make available or utilise the necessary biochemical elements from the diet.

2. Elimination of metabolic wastes and availability of proper nutritional elements are necessary for effective results from manipulative therapy.

3. Manipulative therapy provides a method of stimulating the movement of all body fluids, especially lymph and cerebrospinal fluids, thus giving the cooperating patient additional relief, even if not complete cure.

4. Remember it takes time, patience and cooperation between the patient and their family and doctor in order to obtain maximum results in the treatment of rheumatoid disorders.

## CHRONIC ARTHRITIS

Arthritis may be caused by infection in the cervix or prostate. There are many types of arthritis (such as infective, atrophic or rheumatoid arthritis), which show up as inflammation of the joints. The condition may be systemic, the joint infection being just one manifestation. The treatment to the affected joints can be no more than palliative whilst the infection is still active and not removed – that infection appears in the cervix in arthritic women and the prostate in men. If effectual treatment is applied to these areas and the cause eradicated, the result will be an arrest of arthritis, whether the joints are treated or not. It is well known that cervicitis and prostatitis are forms of pelvic infection.

## DEGENERATIVE, HYPERTROPHIC OR OSTEOARTHRITIS

These are not associated with any form of bacterial toxaemia and no infection is responsible. It was found in some cases that an endocrine imbalance plays some part in its aetiology. When it is due to changes consequent on advancing age, it seems to remain incurable but responds to certain forms of treatment for alleviating pain. The common form is suffered by women and is known as menopausal arthritis, and this is amenable to certain forms of therapy.

## INFECTIVE OR RHEUMATOID ARTHRITIS (IN WOMEN)

It has been recorded that this form is much more common in women than men – it usually occurs during the childbearing period of life, from the ages of 18 to 45. The commonest history is that of ill health either coincident with or preceding the arthritis, perhaps dating back to childbirth or miscarriage, both of which may cause cervicitis. Often the woman dates it to her marriage and perhaps a gonorrhoea infection, which plays a big part. It is also possible that in some cases, especially in virgins, acute specific fevers and also appendicitis are factors in bringing about an infection of the cervix. It has been found clinically that the patient is usually thin, sallow and often anaemic; there may also be slight pyrexia; the joint affection is poly-arthritis, the main brunt being borne by the smaller joints such as the fingers, toes, wrists and ankles, though the large joints are also affected. The arthritis is often symmetrical – the finger-ends are cold and atrophic and often the patient exhibits a peculiar dampness and clamminess of hands and fingers.

The affected joints are swollen and the fingers usually show a fusiform enlargement: this is a characteristic of infective arthritis, whilst nodular enlargements are indicative of osteoarthritis. Joints are usually stiff and movement is painful. There may, in time, be damage to the joints, producing permanent fixation or sometimes splaying of the articular ends due to the pull of the tendons and consequent hypermobility – great deformity is often produced and ulnar deviation of the fingers and bony ankylosis is commonplace.

There is usually abdominal tenderness and the condition of the cervix varies with the stage of the arthritis. It is very common to find some active infection with discharge associated with tenderness in the fornicis. Often, in longstanding cases, the cervix may show only the signs of past infections. It may show a deformity and bear white scars where the infection was healed – often, there are follicles dotted about in its substance, showing that the focus has died out and the arthritis has become dormant.

In many cases of severe arthritis, the only changes X-rays show are the rarefaction of the bone ends, though there may be some diminution of joint space. In some cases the bone adjacent to the joint surfaces is seen to be irregularly arranged and ulcerated and the bone ends contain irregularly arranged areas of rarefaction and sclerosis, the normal lamellar bone structure being destroyed. In many cases, bridges of bone will eventually form across the joint space and cause firm ankylosis.

It has been observed that in most cases of infective arthritis, in the larger joints (the hips, knees and vertebral column) there is usually a formation of inflammatory new bone in the tendons attached to the joints, in the capsules and periarticular structures. This inflammatory new bone is seen as a spur which is usually denser than the normal bone. The true osteophytic growth characteristic of osteoarthritis is usually not denser, but often shows the lamellelate structure of true bone.

### Modes of Onset

There are five distinct modes of onset in women:

1. Usually the joints are found to be affected in two ways – some show up on the X-ray as being destroyed, while others show atrophy of the bones with dislocation. This shows that the fixed joints were affected early and that fixation occurred rapidly. Subsequently, the other joints became involved slowly and insidiously. I feel strongly that these fixed joints are affected by pyaemic process caused by gonorrhoea or puerperal sepsis. The acute process dies out and leaves a form of chronic cervicitis and the resulting toxaemia affects the other joints.

2. Sometimes the joints are involved insidiously, with pain and swelling, leading over the course of years to the patient

becoming a complete cripple. Note that ankylosis does not occur.

3. Rheumatic fever type of onset: it resembles rheumatic fever, with malaise, sweating, pyrexia and fugitive joint pains. The inflammation then settles in one or more joints, showing typical signs of arthritis.

4. In this type, the actual onset of the arthritis is preceded by months or even years of backache and vaginal discharge dating from a confinement or miscarriage. It is commonly termed backache-cervicitis syndrome. It ultimately passes into a state of typical rheumatoid arthritis, the joints being involved one after the other. I must stress that this backache-cervicitis syndrome usually ends in chronic arthritis and one must be able to recognise it. Always regard the backache-cervicitis syndrome as a pre-arthritic condition. I state that chronic arthritis is commonly due to puerperal infection and the effective means of preventing this state would ultimately prevent this form of arthritis.

5. This type is usually associated with the menopause and is often confused with osteoarthritis owing to the age of the patient. The history usually reveals that the patient has suffered with backache and vaginal discharge and that toxaemia has existed in the body for some time. In some cases of infective arthritis, if left untreated, the patient goes steadily downhill – others have frequent remissions.

### Treatment
Focal – this is the same as a pelvic infection and responds to removal of the infective cause. In other words, first remove the cause of infection and then treat the infected joints. Remember that the extent of recovery is in correspondence with the amount of damage done.

## ARTHRITIS IN MEN
1. Infective arthritis is not so common in men as in women. The onset is usually at the age of puberty – there is a difference in the age incidence.

2. Both the cervix and the prostate are equally exposed to

infection by gonorrhoea and other infective factors – cases are therefore rare before puberty. The cervix runs the extra risk of childbirth and miscarriage, though it becomes somewhat atrophied after menopause. Arthritis coming on after the age of 65 is very rare.

3. The prostate often becomes enlarged, degenerate and prone to infection after middle age. Thus a man is more likely to get arthritis after middle age. Sometimes the arthritis is preceded by backache and ill health. The joints don't differ in any way to those of women.

4. Examination of the abdomen usually reveals some tenderness in the lower region, often on one side only. The tender area is usually hyperaesthetic to a pinprick, the sensitive area encircling the body like a half-belt and corresponding to the lower dorsal and upper lumbar segments of the cord.

Examination of the prostate may reveal nothing abnormal, but if the prostate is tender on one side, there will be found a tender area on the abdominal wall on the same side. There may be general prostate tenderness and the gland may feel boggy or hard in one lobe or nodular. Physical signs are variable – microscopic examination of any secretion expressed by massage is not often helpful unless there is infection from gonorrhoea, or it may be only an indication of an excess of leucocytes.

## Modes of Onset
1. Rapid involvement and fixation of few joints followed by slow development of non-ankylosing arthritis in others.

2. Slow insidious onset in all joints affected.

3. The rheumatic fever type of onset, as in women.

4. The backache-prostatitis syndrome (the type called cervicitis in women) this is quite common and most cases start with an attack of gonorrhoea often many years before. The patient suffers from easy fatigue and listlessness with low backache and abdominal pain. Indigestion and other complaints are usually found. Apart from the back pain, the outstanding symptom is nervousness, and these cases are usually labelled neurasthenia. I make sure to examine for prostatitis; the syndrome is a pre-arthritis one.

*Progress*
Follows the same pattern as for women.

*Treatment*
I work to remove the infection of the prostate. Intra-pelvic heating methods have proved valuable.

## OSTEOARTHRITIS

This is usually a form of menopausal syndrome and is amenable to treatment. Normally it is associated with menstrual irregularities and also with hyperthyroidism. It may affect any joint, but usually appears in the larger ones. Normally the weight-bearing joints are affected worst. Joints appear enlarged, probably due to the thickening of periarticular structures. The patient usually complains that the knee locks and then spontaneously recovers and often that the joint lets them down; in that case the joint cavity is usually extended with enlarged synovia. Some ridging of the articular margin can be felt at an early stage and rubbing the patella on the underlying cartilage gives a sensation of roughness – X-rays reveal lipping of bone at the articular margins. This is usually due to some endocrine disturbance.

The beginning and end of adult life is marked by rearrangements in the balance of power between the ductless glands – the total effect of these rearrangements towards the end of life makes up one aspect of what we call senility – and osteoarthritis is a very common manifestation of it. In old age, there is the same liability to this form of arthritis in both sexes. In women, there is a phase of senility at the menopause. The joint infection in women ranges itself with evanescent symptoms of the menopause which, in passing away, leaves the arthritis in an arrested condition. The amount of damage to the joints depends on the length of time the menopause has lasted. Shortening the time lessens the damage. Always remember that mobilisation is always an essential part of all treatments: if you don't use it, you will lose it!

## SPONDYLITIS

There are two types, though its essential characteristics are similar to those of chronic arthritis:

1. *Infective spondylitis or spondylitis ankylopoietica*: caused by cervix

or prostate infection with gonococcal or otherwise. If not due to this, its origin will be found in intestinal or gastric ulceration following dysentery. Intestinal toxaemia is NOT a cause for infective spondylitis or arthritis, unless the lymphatics or intercellular spaces are opened up by ulceration.

2. *Degenerative of decrescent spondylitis or spondylitis deforms*: usually changes made in the vertebral column. Inflammatory changes or calcification occur in these structures. The condition results in pain and great limitation of movement in the spine, the end result being the poker-back spine. This is nearly always associated with inflammatory changes in the sacroiliac joint, which is often affected before the spine. This condition is even more commonly due to prostatic infection. It is said that osteoarthritis of the spine is incurable, but draining of the lymphatics seems to be the main key to all treatments.

### Acupuncture for Arthritis
The most important factor in acupuncture is whether you have touched the correct point or not. If the points are touched and you know from the patient that the energy is passing in the desired direction (in whatever way you want it to pass), then you will see some miracles. Treatment should be once daily if possible, for three to seven minutes: leave the needles in and heat with Moxa. After removing needles, rub the affected areas with the thumb.

On the project I was involved with in Holland, I learned from double-blind trial tests that body, mind and spirit must work together in degenerative diseases for healing to take place, although arthritis is often seen as a physical problem. I saw this clearly with a very pretty young woman who, at the age of 36, developed crippling arthritis. There was a hormonal imbalance present, but problems of rejection in her marriage also surfaced. When I looked at her mental and spiritual state, I got a really good picture and saw that she had tremendous emotional problems. Nevertheless, when I did hormonal balancing using *Optivite* from Lamberts and *Knotgrass Formula* from Bioforce (which is an excellent herbal remedy), it was of great benefit. I also prescribed *Evening primrose* and *Glucosamine*. Taking that combination, she started to get better. For her emotional problems, acupuncture and relaxation treatments did a wonderful job. When I spoke to her again some years later, she reminded me of that very unpleasant time in her life, when she had to overcome her emotional problems before her physical problems started to improve. Luckily, she returned to a happy life and remarried the most wonderful husband she could have wished for. Sometimes, when life is difficult, it is important to remember that behind the clouds there is always sunshine.

In the next two parts of the book, we will learn a little bit more about the mind and the soul, and you will begin to have a much clearer picture of the body as a whole.

# MIND

The mind is a very difficult part of the human body to understand. If everything is in balance, the mind is brilliant. We can compare this to a train, which will stop at every destination when each plug is in the right socket at the signal box. That is a very simple way of describing how the mind works. If the wrong plug is in the wrong socket, problems occur. The most brilliant brains can go from one extreme to the other – Iris Murdoch, the writer who became senile in old age, is a very good example of that. The mind, with its frustrations, fear and other mental states, ends in crystallised matter at the negative pole (pelvic basin).

The energy distribution is carried out by the glandular areas. These, like a spinning wheel, whirl from the right and increase in their circumference, energising the five zones on each side of the body, right and left. The downward thrust constitutes the line which transverses the entire body, both back and front, and so also does the upward thrust. Hence, you have the five lines on each side of the body. Each zone line passes through different portions of the anatomy.

For therapy, the positive, negative and neutral poles are most important, especially the positive, which endeavours to reach the negative. In good health, this is the rhythm of life. Mental upsets, bad eating habits and all the other factors which modern civilisation has thrust upon us obstruct this rhythm in varying degrees. The positive pole is short-circuited, like the fuse box that controls the lighting system. The negative pole (pelvic basin) keeps piling up as a result. Some people are in varying degrees of ill health, with acute and chronic states. The life-giving energy is also locked in varying degrees – when this gets blocked entirely, death is the result.

## TENSIONS

When people talk glibly about tension, they are really only thinking of mental tension. A muscle is capable of contraction and relaxation. In muscular spasm, the blood is squeezed out of the spastic muscle and oxygen cannot get to the tissues. Nature then gives its warning, which we call 'pain'.

It is an established fact that everything in nature is in a state of molecular tension – nothing stands still, for stillness is death and destruction. Tension is a natural state of being and its function. It is the most important factor in physical life – it is responsible for the birth of form, controlling the harmonious distribution of energy through the body. It is this state of tension that preserves the integrity of form. The molecular construction of anything, be it animate or inanimate, is very dependent on this natural law. Call it life, health, energy or what you will, tension is the factor that keeps molecules from flying off into space. The tensile strength of a human cell is an electrical phenomena and is allied to its frequency or rate of vibration. When this is altered by unhealthy living, the frequency and tension is altered. The end result is disease and disharmony.

Tension, as we know it, is muscular in nature, whether it be produced by the cold weather (we automatically tense ourselves), emotional stimuli or other factors. We know what happens when a muscle remains in a state of tension for any length of time.

Inner conflict and emotional upsets are what cause most functional diseases and these factors, when persistent, actually precipitate soluble calcium from the bloodstream into the joints. Mind has thus become matter and the results are arthritis, rheumatism, lumbago and other illnesses. This is called the 'negative miracle'. The 'positive miracle' is to supplant the latter by such tendencies as joy, happiness and other ideal conditions for survival.

The contraction of muscles is due to nerve impulses passing to the muscle via a spinal nerve trunk to the nerve endings of the muscle. In a normal person, this contraction, followed by relaxation (mainly in exercise), improves the metabolism and also increases the circulation of the blood, which flows through the muscle ensuring that it receives strength. When the nerves, through disease or injury, are no longer able to conduct these nerve impulses, in most cases muscle contraction becomes impossible. When a muscle remains contracted, the result is fatigue, pain and other harmful effects. Its supply of oxygen is cut off and the blood and lymph are also squeezed out of the tissues affected. What happens is that the fibres making up the muscles contract violently, but fail to relax properly, so that the blood and oxygen are prevented from reaching the muscle. This stress state is considered by many medical doctors to end in muscle spasm. Factors like worry, fear and anxiety can bring on tension in muscles and this leads to the names given to diseases such as fibrositis, neuritis etc.

It is generally not known that cases like asthma are also due to a spasm which, when the lungs are about to evacuate the air inhaled, prevents expiration by dilating the alveoli of the lungs and contracting the bronchial tubes. This complaint makes the life of the sufferer real martyrdom. Angina pectoris is essentially also caused by a spasm which obstructs the coronary arteries, the arteries which convey food and oxygen to the cardiac muscles, so that the blood can no longer reach the tissues of the body.

It is well worth making a mental note that the sympathetic nervous system reaches all organs and controls blood circulation to all parts. Also, the nervous system controls all muscular effort and the stimulation of the ganglion of Impar and the perineum techniques are the key.

Muscle spasm pulls the tendons, ligaments and bones, throwing them out of alignment. Just replacing or correcting a misaligned bone is merely a palliative move, for these corrections never stay put for long. No matter what the condition, be it lumbago, slipped discs, rheumatism, torticollis or female complaints, the release of the muscles, in a spasmodic state, must be the focus.

Going still deeper into this very important and interesting factor, the cerebrospinal and the sympathetic chain nerves are joined together by the vagus (positive and negative), linking the conscious and subconscious minds. All anxiety neuroses turn the urine alkaline. You can prove this for yourself by testing. When there is too much alkalinity, it paves the way for disease in the body. Bacteria of all strains flourish in an alkaline base. All tensions, frustrations, fears, phobias and repressions tend to create excessive alkalinity over a period of time. In other words, with negative thoughts, you change the frequency of the wavelength of the normal cell structure within the organism. Added to this, we eat too much protein, keeping the human body in continual high gear – the rat race demands this in these modern, 'civilised' times.

Where does this lead us? An easy and almost miraculous way to offset all these problems is to stimulate the positive and negative ends of the sympathetic chain or ganglion. When a positive thought is held for long enough, it is propelled by the cosmic law of attraction to the negative, or material, plane and becomes a reality to the person who has formulated it. In other words, it sends a message to the body cells, affecting them in a positive way. The cells of the body hold physical memories of both positive and negative thoughts; likewise, the positive and negative ends of the sympathetic chain. The positive and negative are stimulated and the break or fuse affecting the organism is repaired. Harmony exists once again. Thus, the triangle is complete – the positive, negative and neutral are in balance.

Always keep in mind, during your treatments, that the artery rules supreme through the sympathetic nervous system, as the circulation flows supplying the body's needs, with or without us being really conscious of it. Only when the sympathetic nervous system is functioning properly can the spine stimulate the natural function of the body.

## THE NERVOUS SYSTEM

'As man thinketh, so shall he be.'

Stiff muscles are nearly always due to impeded venous circulation of the blood, or to the irritation of the nervous system, causing the muscular fibres to contract around nerve filaments and increasing the muscular contraction.

Disease is a condition of undue pressure (interference with normal conditions, such as muscular contraction). It is an undisputable fact that when the nervous system is permitted to perform its normal function, disease cannot exist in the body. All bodily functions are performed through the nervous system, making it imperative that one should fully understand its workings and function. When the nervous system is unduly interfered with, disharmony ensues. This denominates a diseased condition – as soon as harmony is restored, the disease ceases to exist. The theme should be 'take off the pressure', for then all is free, nature is satisfied and friction ceases. Since muscular contraction is the cause of nerve pressure and the interference of nerve function, relaxation becomes a necessity to permit the normal flow of fluids through the vessels.

To know the condition is of more importance than the diagnosis, or the name of a disease. The nervous system pervades every part of the human body and the functions of the five senses. Always remember that the nervous system is the media through which all functions are performed. Insomuch as normal tissue is a product of nerve influence and function, the mind through the nerve filaments has the entire supervision of the body. It is rational to conclude that, to relieve any abnormal condition, it would be of primary importance to free the nervous system from all obstruction.

All rational human beings act as they think, hence all actions are the product of thought (excluding accidents and trauma). It is rational to assume that disease is also a product of thought. If disease was natural, then it would be wrong to use any means to relieve the person afflicted with disease. Nature heals from within.

The nervous system secretes pneumogastric acids. The splanchnic nervous system (from the fifth to twelfth dorsal) manufactures alkaline secretions (liver secretions, pancreas). A spinal adjustment or manipulation anywhere between these dorsals neutralises an excess which may prevail in either of the two departments controlled by the pneumogastric or splanchnic.

There are many things a person can do for themselves, such as breathe, eat, sleep, exercise and think properly. All of these are part of treatment and will help relieve many conditions thought of as disease.

The vasomotor area is of primary importance. When the system is freed, the arterial circulation is regulated and the capillaries are filled with healthy blood. The sympathetic system superintends the digestion process and should not be diverted. As all the secretions along the alimentary canal are superintended by the mind, through the nervous system, it is very important that it be allowed to finish the digestion before being directed elsewhere.

Disease is only a condition. Every doctor and practitioner should study the nature of each condition to be remedied. The object of the treatment should always be to remove nerve pressure and allow freedom of fluid circulation, and freedom from muscular contractures. These objectives are to be accomplished by the treatment given, whatever the modality may be.

Bacteria plays little part in producing disease: all pathological conditions are the result of impeded venous circulation and bacteria only invades where decomposition has already taken place.

The pneumogastric system has the special function of generating acid secretions in the body and the splanchnic nervous system has the opposite function of generating an alkaline secretion. I prefer to designate these as the positive (yang) and negative (yin) forces. The balance of yin and yang determines the state of health and well-being.

Excessive activity of the pneumogastric system produces too much acidity. Excessive acid in the blood causes irritation of the nervous system. Then contractures of muscle tissues and venous stasis follow and toxaemia ensues. Should the secretion be excessively alkaline, a tissue disturbance known as dyscrasia (a depraved or abnormal state) will usually result. This will then lead to a tendency to boils, tumours, etc. Make a mental note that the pneumogastric and the splanchnic form what is known as 'the solar plexus'.

## THE PINEAL GLAND
The pineal gland is the governing gland of the entire body and the seat of the superconscious mind. Very little is known about the superconscious mind – it is in constant contact with our own creation. The pituitary gland is secondary to it and coordinates all the other glands. The glandular impulses set by radiations or fields of either positive (yang) or negative (yin) qualities form the body's rays, commonly called the 'aura'. Always remember that when the fluid wave of the brain is disturbed, the vibratory rate of the glands or the auras are affected. This changes the nerve flow impulses and the negative and positive balance. The next change is chemical and the next is glandular imbalance.

## STRESS
Take any average person, on any corner of any busy street. It is easy to get the impression that a very high percentage of people are sick, because they do not display a happy, relaxed, smiling countenance. Some look worried, tired and pale. Some seem to have a bent posture. Some appear to be gasping for breath. Others appear agitated and excited, while some look apathetic, resigned to the surrounding environment and allowing

themselves to be pushed around. Many accept these conditions as normal living. They go through life hurrying and scurrying day in, day out. Some of them will eventually call on their doctor and admit that they suffer aches and pains, that their bodies are lacking in efficiency or that they have hidden fears and anxieties.

Pain and discomfort are manifested through the medium of the nerves and their centres, of which there are two sets of systems: the cerebrospinal nervous system and the autonomic nervous system. The former deals almost exclusively with the physical body, the functions of the five senses and the voluntary, objective functions of the body, and has to do with pathology. The autonomic nervous system deals with the involuntary and subjective, influencing psychosomatic diseases. Someone may show no pathological signs of disease (none of the obvious alterations usually related to illness) and yet may suffer pain and discomfort, and be truly sick, for disturbing nerve impulses or vibrations are being transmitted to their physical body. If these negative nerve impulses are replaced with positive, healthy impulses and vibrations full of vital energy, the body assumes a normal, healthy state. This can be achieved through positive thought. In the final part of this book, a meditation specifically for this purpose is given.

The disturbing negative cellular impulses originate, in most cases, in a patient's own mind. Psychosomatic sickness is brought about through wrong or poisonous thought. What happens is that our mental state influences the psychic body and through the sympathetic nervous system transmits negative vibrations to the physical body, causing aches and pains. It would be safe to say that in about 85 per cent of cases, no pathology, or actual cause of disease, is found.

Now, what about diseases where there *is* definite pathology? Here, too, in a great many cases, the causes are the same. The patient's anxieties and insecurities, total ignorance of the simple general principles in life, fear of pain and death, or of loss of power and influence, may become an illness which eventually manifests as pathological changes in the body. It is possible to break out in definite, visible changes. The term so commonly used, 'to break out in a rash', is not without basic truth. Have you never gone red in the face when excited, or turned pale and broken into a sweat when frightened? Eczema and asthma, nausea and vomiting, indigestion and stomach (or duodenal) ulcers, high blood pressure and heart disease, arthritis and crippling body deformities, sterility and miscarriages, and a score of other illnesses can be attributed directly to one's mental state.

A very common ailment, which is widespread and prevalent among busy executives, is stomach ulcers. Emotional tension stimulates the glands of the stomach to secrete more acid than normally required. This excessive acid will then start digesting and burning the delicate stomach lining. This carries on *ad infinitum* and can eventually end in cancer. Remove the emotional strain and the ulcers will clear up.

When treating a patient medicine is not enough, even though remarkable advances in medical science have done a tremendous service to humankind in prolonging life and helping eliminate disease. We can give a patient antacids and even operate and remove the secreting glands, but we cannot – with medicine alone – promise a permanent cure. This method does not remove the mental factor and sometimes even aggravates it.

Mental functions are only a part of our general physical make-up. A practitioner who convinces a patient that their mental state and emotional upsets may be causing their disease, and who can influence them to change their mental attitudes, will undoubtedly go far towards helping that patient cure his illness. But even that is not enough. Recognising the mental factor as the cause of disease is recognising only the physical, or negative, side of man and only half the problem. Happiness lies in the positive half, the soul and its affinity to the cosmos. Mental fixations can be very stubborn and deeply ingrained in one's mind. They can form a permanent block to successful treatment and good health. To overcome this block, the psychic body has to be activated into its normal and rightful function.

Modern science teaches us that nature operates under intelligent laws and that all actions of the objects of nature are intelligent actions. Mind is the power which can react through the physicality of the environment. It makes natural relations orderly and is the source of universal harmony that keeps the stars on their courses and makes the earth bloom in the summer and sleep in the winter, which makes us who we are and sustains us through strife and turmoil, and heals our ills and mends our broken hearts when life has been too hard.

The mind acting is the mind thinking; the product of thinking is thought. In other words, an action of the mind is a thought, and the process of mind-acting is thinking. All thoughts, whether conscious or unconscious, are expressed, but many of them are expressed only in the organisms of the thinker. It is necessary to have a means by which to convey thoughts from one person to another. Language is such a means and the organic process of using language for the conveyance of thought from one person to another is called speech. There are, of course, many forms of speech – the spoken word is not the only one, it is not even the one most frequently used. The use of the hands is a form of speech, and is most effective. The mind needs no word to command the hands.

In solving a mathematical problem, a recognition of the principle involved is the only means by which one may arrive at the correct solution – so too with the problem of health. To recognise and apply the principle underlying the individual life constitutes the metaphysical solution to this vital question. When you become conscious of principle (and there are varying degrees of this consciousness) you enter into closer mental touch with the principle.

Faith is the key to emancipation from every ill and every wrong: faith in self, in God and humankind. It is the secret of all real accomplishment and great achievement. There is nothing that inspires, uplifts and heals so much as faith when combined with love.

## PHYSICAL SIGNS OF DISEASE

The Ancients have left many gems for us to seek, learn and apply. I was taught to look, to listen and to feel. With this in mind, here are some sure indicators that will help you to a conclusion of applying the right treatment.

When we grow old, the white at the bottom of our eyes shows. Adults with the white showing are in a very negative condition. Their organs are weakened and, having little reflex ability in case of danger, they are prone to accidents.

Blinking very often signifies the body's attempt to discharge excess negative energy in any way it can. One should not blink one's eyes more than three times per minute.

A prominent red colour in the whites of the eyes is a sign of a bad liver. The liver has grown tired due to an over-consumption of food, especially animal produce. When the red has spread all over the whites of the eye, the organs are malfunctioning.

If the eyes move constantly or are slow to react (to follow

your finger), there is a problem with the heart; its pace is not normal. In such cases, the pupil will be too big. A moon on the top part of the iris or a white ring around it indicates malfunctioning in the abdominal area.

Swelling around the eyes, particularly a swelling of the upper eyelid, indicates gallstones. When the stones pass, the swelling drops immediately. A dark-brown colour under the eyes indicates excessively positive kidneys and trouble in the female organs.

Swelling under the eyes indicates kidney stones. A formation of gallstones or blood stagnation may also be indicated.

Dark blue or violet under the eyes reveals blood stagnation, probably caused by an over-consumption of fruit, sugar and meat.

Bulging eyes indicate a negative condition and thyroid trouble.

Pimples on the interior of the eyelid signify excess protein. They usually appear and disappear relatively quickly.

An eyelid that is almost white signifies anaemia. The inside of the eyelid should be red. To examine, gently pinch the eyelid and pull it away from the eye.

A broad, thick eyebrow is positive. A thin eyebrow is negative. Too much sweet food, especially sugar, makes the eyebrows thinner and eventually causes them to disappear. People with almost no eyebrows are prone to cancer.

An examination of the nose can tell much about the condition of the person being diagnosed. Reduce your intake of food and you will see your nose grow smaller. Your nose can save your life because it gives so much away. A long nose starting high up on the face is negative. A short nose indicates a strong constitution. A small nose pointing upwards is a sign of strong, positive energy.

The centre of the nose indicates the condition of the heart. An enlarged nose shows an enlarged heart (the result of excessive eating and drinking). The nostrils show the condition of the lungs: the larger the better. Small nostrils indicate weak lungs. Well-developed nostrils are a sign of masculinity. A fat nose, which is somewhat oily and shiny, indicates over-consumption of animal protein. Red vessels on the tip of the nose are an indication of high blood pressure and a sign that heart disease will follow.

A small mouth is positive. A large mouth is negative. A

horizontal line between the mouth and nose shows a malfunctioning of the sexual organs. The lips should be of equal thickness. In general, thick lips indicate a positive constitution and thin lips a negative constitution. The size of the upper lip shows the condition of the liver. If the lip is swollen, the liver is enlarged, the subject eats too much and is prone to mental disorders. The size of the lower lip indicates the condition of the large intestine. When the lower lip is swollen, there is a weakness and looseness in the intestines, and therefore constipation. Epilepsy is a possibility when both lips are enlarged. This condition indicates that, as a child, the patient was given too much food.

Lips should usually be pink, although they grow darker with age. A young person with dark lips has blood stagnation. Their blood circulation is bad due to an excessive intake of animal protein and strongly negative foods. People with dark lips tend to develop cancer, pineal troubles and diseases of the sexual organs.

The texture of the lips reveals the condition of the stomach. A cyst on the right side of the mouth indicates stomach trouble, acidity or the beginning of an ulcer on the left side of the stomach. A cyst on the left side of the mouth indicates a problem in the right side of the stomach.

A wide chin denotes strong kidneys. A narrow, pointed chin denotes kidney disease.

Pale cheeks with red spots indicate intestinal disorders. Extreme paleness of the cheeks means intestinal inactivity.

Dry, thin lips mean the glands are under-active. Thin, pale lips are a sign of frigidity.

When the mammary glands are functioning poorly the lips are usually straight and have no downward curve. The mother will seldom nurse her offspring.

Fullness, redness and a moist centre of the upper lip means a strong reproductive system; the reverse means a weak reproductive system.

A broad, high forehead, fine skin, hair and bright eyes, with the ears well forward, denote a well-developed nervous system and brain.

The strength of the spine is denoted by the length of the upper lip. A short upper lip means a weak column.

The longer the septum of nose, the better the liver is developed and able to fulfil its work. A short septum indicates the reverse.

Large nostrils denote healthy, strong lungs and also a strong heart and muscular system.

If the bridge of the nose is broad and high, this normally indicates a strong, well-functioning stomach.

Large, convex eyes denote a well-developed system.

## THE SYMPATHETIC NERVOUS SYSTEM

Pottinger and others have stated that every internal organ, gland and tissue has either a direct or reflex connection with the surface of the body. It has already been mentioned that the artery (blood) reigns supreme. Simply stated, this means the blood is kept in circulation by rhythmic contraction of the vessel walls.

The heart, arterioles, arteries, veins and vasomotor system exist and function in order that they may perform the service of distribution and elimination. The arteriole, the capillary and the vasomotor system are an important part of the system we call the 'effector mechanism'.

Whatever affects the nervous system affects the circulatory system to the same degree. It is worth noting that the nervous system is the organiser of all experience and is also the coordinator of that experience. The nervous system is not a disease-producing entity, but a system arranged to coordinate the many functions of the body. Whilst it is true that some somatic nerves carry sympathetic and parasympathetic fibres and also convey some of the vasomotor signals to their destination, the main function of the nervous system is to conduct sensory impulses to the brain, and motor impulses back to the area for motor action.

The autonomic nervous system is divided into several parts, the first of these being the sympathetic nervous system. It is responsible for holding the normal, plastic tone of the organs. Any increase in tone above the norm is capable of producing pain. There is no pain in the absence of tension.

I do not wish to burden you with minute details of the origins and ultimate destination of the nerves. It is enough to say that the sympathetic nervous system affects the whole system in some way. Affecting the sympathetics also involves the parasympathetics. The system is arranged in such a manner that it is possible to maintain life and regulate function regardless of what may happen to the spine below the fifth dorsal.

We have the vasodilators and vasoconstrictors within this system. To elucidate, we shall call them the vasomotors of the sympathetic origin and vasomotors the of the parasympathetic origin. Simply stated, everything exists for the benefit of the cell and thus it also exists for the benefit of the arteriole and the capillary.

Using the nasal probe technique, the plexuses become sensitive to changes in blood pressure, changes in blood temperature and the circulation of the bloodstream. All this and much more is due to the irritation of the nasal mucosa. This is very important in terms of the reflexes. These methods can affect the pituitary gland, so it will be appreciated that the emotions can be greatly helped due to their close connection with this gland.

## THE FIVE LAWS OF LIFE

1. *Oxidisation.* Oxidisation is the keystone of health. Life is in the blood. Oxygen is the bridge between life and death, between health and disease.

2. *Elimination.* Removal of waste. The accumulation of waste in the body with its toxic by-products could kill you in 24 hours.

3. *Nutrition.* The building and repair of body. The energy to function is maintained by the use of oxygen in the tissues.

4. *Motion.* Or vibration, expansion and contraction of cells, muscles and tissues.

5. *Relaxation.* Rest. The least expenditure of energy still keeps the body functioning.

The blood is purified by oxygen in the lungs. Everyone with ill health lacks enough blood oxygen. No bacteria can live in pure oxygen or pure blood. If the respiratory tract is obstructed in any manner, oxygen starvation results, leading to disease in the open cavities of the nose, throat and ears, and also in the closed cavities elsewhere in the body.

## THE FIVE MOST IMPORTANT FUNCTIONS OF OXYGEN

1. It has combustible units of gas that give off heat. These units

of heat make soluble nutritional elements fit for absorption in the body.

2. The vapour that keeps the gas in solution has a dissolving power greater than any other element entering the body. This moisture, combined with heat, melts secretions and renders them liquid for elimination.

3. Oxygen attracts iron to the body. This is one of the essential elements for stamina and virility.

4. Oxygen maintains cell rate activity.

5. Oxygen is an aid to the sinuses for balance in the body and resonance of the voice.

Almost all bacterial diseases mean a patient is lacking in oxygen; the functions of oxygen in the open cavities of the head and the closed cavities of the body are necessary to health.

Oxidation is life − you can be paralysed and live, but you cannot live without oxygen, no matter how many adjustments you make. The process of exchange of carbon dioxide for oxygen is continuous, ending only at death. The rate of exchange may be fast or slow.

## BRAIN REFLEXES
There are numerous methods of affecting the brain through treatment directed towards the movement of cranial bones. We have only to place our hands upon various portions of the skull to feel this slight movement upon swallowing, yawning, crying, sneezing and even talking. Usually the movement that is felt and heard is remote from the area under treatment.

If we study the articulation of the cranial bones which guard the cranial vault, particularly at the sutures, we observe that they are designed to resist pressure from the outside − the more pressure applied from the outside, the faster these bones lock. Pressure from outside tends to lock the bones in their position, while the intercranial pressure tends to loosen or unlock them. Basically, we have two reasons for treating the cranium: firstly, to equalise the circulation and pressure of the spinal fluid and, secondly, to stimulate or normalise the various intercranial centres into activity.

The hypothalamus and the thalamus are both functional units. Each of these structures plays its own part in the perfect coordination of sensory stimuli. These structures are the end organs of the sensory nervous system. The simple act of disturbance by movement of the spinal fluid sometimes has an immediate and intensive reaction. The increase or decrease of pressure produces a reaction, from negative to positive. Some patients become exhilarated, whilst others fall rapidly to sleep.

Anything that occupies space or interferes with the electrical or magnetic conduction of the brain is capable of producing coma, spasm or even epileptic seizures. Disturbance of the function of the reticular formation or any of its nuclei can, and does, interfere with emotional balance. Psychosis, neurosis, depression and all other mental and personality changes involve the affector mechanism of the sensory system (the reticular formation).

In discussing the subject of brain reflexes, we quickly become conscious of our ignorance. So little is really known of the physiology of the brain. In order to excite and control brain reflexes, we must not depend upon the arteriole pulse as a guide. We must use enough pressure on the designated area to produce a semi-anaemia of the minute blood vessels. This anaemia is sufficient stimulus to produce some cerebral action.

There is a neuro-vascular reflex which is related to an organ and these are located mainly on the human skull. Most of these require a simple pressure associated with a slight stretching of the area involved. This operation will involve a corresponding increase in the circulation of the associated organ.

It is feasible and possible to influence numerous conditions by working on certain areas of the cranium, which will affect the zones of the Rolandic and Sylvian fissures. Areas that are anterior and posterior to the middle portion of the Sylvian fissure are becoming more and more effective in their use.

From the mid portion of the Sylvian fissure, we can contact and affect the nuclei of the midbrain. It is possible to produce speech in an individual who has never spoken, as a result of a birth accident. Hearing may be restored from the same area. While working with the brain reflexes with an adequate stimulus, we may influence the vasomotor centres in the medulla from any area of the cranium. This vasomotor centre is closely allied to the respiratory centre. Therefore, the instance in which

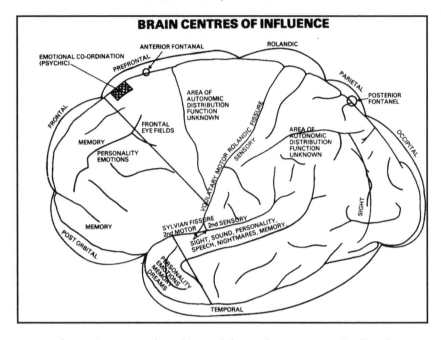

**BRAIN CENTRES OF INFLUENCE**

the patient stops breathing whilst under treatment is directly associated with extreme elevation of temperature on the surface of the head. As long as the respiration, pulse and blood pressure are normal, nothing can happen.

Highly emotional people will often start crying while the emotional centres are under treatment. This is an emotional release and for the good. Every bit of tension is out of the body; even normal plastic tone is reduced. The great miracle that occurs as far as the patient is concerned is a great sense of mental and physical release, with complete comfort. Areas of the skull, when properly and skilfully treated, will produce tremendous brain-centre activity.

The two frontal emotional centres are located upon the frontal bone at the prominent bulges, one on either side. Two centres lie one on either side, just above the zygomatic ridge. These are the temporal tips. They affect the emotional centres which lie within the tips of the temporal lobes of the brain. The third pair lies in the midsylvian area of the brain. Its location on the skull lies on a line drawn upwards from the front of the ear to a point which would bisect the temporal sutures. The area is very small, so one must be exact. Anterior to the midsylvian area lies the secondary motor area to the brain and posterior to this point lies the secondary sensory areas. The entire midsylvian area is no larger than a ten-pence piece.

Associated with these areas is an aspect of behaviour, the elusive thing called personality. The emotional centres of the brain are closely associated with each other. The frontal centres are most often disturbed as a result of emotional factors involving the upper digestive system. The tension diseases involving these centres find expression in gall bladder disease, gastric and duodenal ulcers, pancreatitis and other illnesses.

The vasomotor system controls the blood vessels and is located in the medulla. It controls the diameter of the arterioles and capillaries of the skin and subcutaneous tissue. The ability to do this and influence effector mechanisms is a powerful approach to both the nervous system and the circulatory system. The vasomotor nervous system is a go-between, or catalyst, between the sensory and motor systems of the body.

The senses provide a stimulus which arises either in the spinal recticular system or in the recticular system of the brain stem. Before any motor activity can take place, vasodilation must take place in that part of the cortex that corresponds to the part to be actuated.

The autonomic nervous system functions in a metabolic way, but the vasomotor nervous system functions in the capillary bed. There is a parallel pattern with the vasomotor reflex to the muscle, and an intimate relationship between the various centres on the skull and muscles, just as there is an intimate relationship between the vasomotor system and the muscles. The vasomotor system, the lymphatic nervous system and the cerebral spinal fluid all interact and interrelate, and reflexes affecting one affect the other, but often implementation of the vasomotor achieves a faster and speedier result than would be attained otherwise.

Here is a point worth remembering: the vasomotor centres, which control the circulation, are basically the aortic sinus – the two carotid sinuses at the bifurcation of the carotid artery and the next is the point anterior to the coccyx. These vasomotor centres are hooked up with the receptors. If there is a disturbance of function – a slight pressure applied to the aortic sinus (midway, midline on the sternum) along with a contact at the carotid sinus and a slight rectal contact – these are very important reflexes in promoting general circulation and function in treating vasospastic states. Contact the fissure of

Rolando area and also the midsylvian area, and watch the wonderful response.

## THE CEREBROSPINAL SYSTEM
The brain is the great coordinator of all the bodily functions. It does not recognise disease as such, but only views it as an altered function, so all the defensive mechanisms are brought into play to reduce that function. At present, we may affect beneficially any voluntary structure which is not functioning properly, such as the emotions, changes in personality, speech, coordinated vision, some types of epilepsy, multiple sclerosis, cerebral accidents and a host of other conditions wherein a part of the picture may be of cerebral origin or show its effects upon the brain.

The next most important areas are the fontanelles, anterior and posterior. The movement of spinal fluid is, to a great extent, dependent on good diaphragmatic action, and good action of the dome may be brought by treating the fontanelles. While working with the fontanelles, you will find that the patient relaxes rapidly and achieves a degree of comfort. The pulse also becomes soft, long and full, and a full movement of the diaphragm is noticeable. Treatment of the fontanelles is the only treatment given in acute and chronic polio. Good respiration with normal movement of spinal fluid are the two principal things accomplished by treatment of the two fontanelles.

The next centre of importance is the parietal eminence. This area affects the tone of the gastrointestinal tract, from the stomach to the ileo-caecal valve. These parietal lobes of the brain exercise control over the normal plastic tone of the intestines.

The next areas have to do with the drainage of the eye. These areas are known as the 'frontal eye fields'. These lie on either side of the midline of the skull, about an inch to an inch and a half lateral to the midline and about an inch behind the hairline. Treatment of these centres causes a softening and drainage of the eyeball and, at the same time, aids the Muller muscle to return to its normal tone. It is an important area for treatment and relief of glaucoma.

Another area of importance is the one known as the kidney centre. Kidney function influences the pituitary gland and in turn this centre of the brain has an influence on kidney function. Treatment on this point on the skull causes the reflex point on the cartilage of the eighth rib to disappear. The point on the eighth rib is the diagnostic point for kidney dysfunction. The centre produces a change in the urine.

The cerebellum may be affected by treatment on the occipital prominence. The next point lies immediately below the posterior fontanelle, just to the left of the midline of the skull. This is a powerful area for treatment of women in the menopause, as it helps to quieten the symptoms that take place at this time of life.

A very important area (and one that has already been mentioned) is the fissure of Rolando. Lying within the folds of the fissure is a branch of the middle cerebral artery. This is a favourable area for vascular spasms which dramatically produce sudden paralysis (little strokes) and it is also the area we find subdural haemorrhage. One may favourably affect paralysis originating from this area. After locating the Rolandic fissure, move downwards towards the ear, about an inch to an inch and a half along the fissure on the opposite side of the paralysis. Exert your pressure on that exact point for ten to fifteen minutes. As a general rule, cerebral spasms located here are of a flaccid nature, with no spastic element. Vasospasms of haemorrhage may also occur in other areas of the brain which could produce flaccid paralysis. Remember to locate and treat the Rolandic fissure on the opposite cortex, the so-called 'trial and error' method. In any case, the blood pressure must be watched very carefully. With emotional shock and fainting, treatment must be directed toward the normalisation of the pressure of spinal fluid through the fontanelles.

The spinal fluid occupies a number of spaces which may be divided into an inner and outer circulating system. The manner of spinal fluid circulation is not clear – clinically it would seem that respiration is the motive power behind it. Treatment directed toward the fontanelles increases diaphragmatic action, so that respiration becomes smoother and deeper, and increases the flow of spinal fluid.

Let us view the brain as an organ which, when properly coordinated, produces what is known as normal function. It must also be viewed as an organ capable of dysfunction through the medium of glandular changes, nutritional factors, emotional factors and physical influence.

## CRANIAL REFLEX CONTACT POINTS

1. Frontal emotional: this is a gastric reflex and is located on the prominent bulges on each side of the frontal bone. It is related to the stomach and is very good for disturbances of the circulation. This point also affects emotions and stress.

2. Temporal: these two centres lie on either side of the face and just above the zygomatic ridge. These two points work well in emotional tension, together with Number 12.

3. Posterior fontanelle: this point has much to do with body structure. It is located at the posterior fontanelle and is associated with adrenal function. It has a very relaxing effect on the spinal fluid and motion of the diaphragm. Helps respiration and normal fluid movement and can be used in conjunction with the anterior fontanelle, Number 6.

4. Menopausal (glandular): located just below the posterior fontanelle to the left of the midline. It is termed the glandular vasomotor area and also the climacteric area (both male and female). It is associated with glandular activity and affects posture, structure and function.

5. Cerebellum: these two points are located on either side of the occipital protuberance. The cerebellum is a very powerful kidney reflex and also affects the pituitary gland. It is an area of great importance. The cerebellum can also be affected by pressure on the occipital protuberance.

6. Anterior fontanelle: this is located in the anterior fontanelle area and directly affects the lungs. It has a great influence on the diaphragm and the spinal fluids. It is a very important point in chest infections and is also concerned with the posterior fontanelle in affecting body structure.

7. Frontal eye fields: these points are located on either side of the midline of the skull, approximately one and a half inches to either side of the midline and about one inch behind the hairline. This area is concerned with the drainage of the eyes. It is associated with the liver and gall bladder. It has proved useful in cases of glaucoma and other eye complaints.

8. Fissure of Rolando: this is located at the fissure of Rolando

(bilateral). It has a direct effect on the cerebral blood vessels and is very useful in vasospasm or strokes. Either point can be used, depending on which side has been affected. It is very good in cases of paralysis affecting the speech and various forms of aphasia. Remember that the opposite sides are affected. Normally there is no response if the involved area has a haemorrhage.

9. Parietal: located on the points of the parietal eminence. These points directly affect the tone of the gastrointestinal tract, from the gastric area right down to the ileo-caecal valve. Very good contact for abdominal ptosis. All in all, these parietal contacts exercise control over the normal plastic tone of the intestines.

10. Vagus (Vagal): the vagal area is located close to the fissure of Rolando, slightly below. It is associated with vagal function, the pancreas and the second unit of digestion. This point is very effective for both hyper- and hypo-insulinism.

11. Midsylvian (emotional): this point is about the size of a ten-pence piece and is located in the midsylvian area. It is a very important psychosomatic reflex. It is an area for emotional stress and will prove helpful in both sensory and motor function. Very good for use with hypochondriacs and highly emotional people. Treatment here affects 11 other areas.

12. Temporal emotional: located at the point marked on the chart and is always involved with emotional tension and disturbances of the eyes and ears. An elevated occiput and a depressed shoulder surely points to an emotional disturbance.

13. Kidney: this point is shown on the chart and can be used to great advantage. It affects both the pituitary and the kidneys.

## THE ENDOCRINE GLANDS
Our bodies can be compared to a car. There are two conditions for its efficient operation: firstly, the machinery must be in good working order and, secondly, it must be supplied with suitable fuel. Taking this metaphor a little further, in the body the endocrines are similar in function to carburettors, and the autonomic system to the tuning and wiring systems. It is a sorry fact that very little is known or

recorded on the subject of endocrine function and malfunction. It is the lifeline of the human system and, if understood and the knowledge applied, the path to alleviating many symptoms would be in our grasp.

There are physical methods of influencing the endocrines through the feet and also vital areas in the cranial vault. It has long been a misconception that the chakras control the endocrine, but nothing is further from the truth. The chakras circulate the polarity energy to every part of the human body. In so doing, they nourish the energies of the endocrine system, but these chakras are *not* the endocrine system.

### A Few Things to Note and Remember

- The result of motion is the production of energy.
- If a gland has energy and vibration, it is active.
- Every gland serves as a specific workshop or laboratory for the preparation of certain substances. These enter the bloodstream and are utilised to maintain the integrity of the body.
- The endocrine glands represent balance in the body.
- The parotid gland controls the endocrine.
- The physical activity of a person is greatly dependent upon their body chemistry. This is controlled and regulated by the endocrine glands.

## THE ENDOCRINE SYSTEM

The endocrine system exists for the purpose of maintaining the correct state of blood protein and tissue colloids.

- The emotions activate the adrenals.
- The adrenals act on the nervous system.
- The nervous system affects the sympathetics.
- The adrenals link into the thyroid and parasympathetics.

The mechanism of control for healthful function in the body consists of the pituitary-hypothalamus complex: the pituitary supervises and influences the glandular system, while the hypothalamus supervises and influences the autonomic system. The hypothalamus is sensory.

The brain holds in the thalamus a fluid which gives balance to the head, like a spirit level. It is a form of blood plasma and

flows over the nervous system. Comprehension begins in the
pineal gland and thalamus. The suprarenals produce cortin and
adrenalin. They use calcium to build red fibre, nerve and bone
tissue. This gives tone to every cell and strength to the organs. If
there is a weakness and lack of tone, there is a fast, small, weak
pulse, a weak heart muscle, uterine inertia and prolapsed
conditions, auto-intoxication from lack of liver tone, flaccid
constipation and any condition showing lack of tone and low
blood pressure.

In hypofunction, there exists thinness, nervousness, fatigue
and exhaustion, and the patient is always tired. Look for
Addison's disease – a progressive anaemia leading to brown
discolouration of the skin. Normalise the external secretion of
the suprarenals (whichever is slow), for Addison's disease is due
to a hypofunction of the cortex which produces cortin, because
of the medullary or internal function. The medullary secretes
adrenalin and increases the heartbeat as well as the blood
pressure. It inhibits peristalsis, increases metabolism and kidney
function, dilates the pupil, contracts the blood vessels and
shortens coagulation time, and stimulates the smooth muscles.

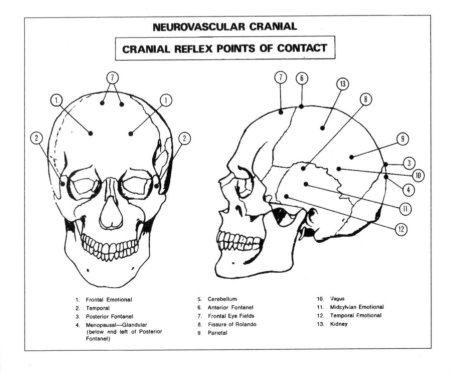

**NEUROVASCULAR CRANIAL**

**CRANIAL REFLEX POINTS OF CONTACT**

| | | |
|---|---|---|
| 1. Frontal Emotional | 5. Cerebellum | 10. Vagus |
| 2. Temporal | 6. Anterior Fontanel | 11. Midsylvian Emotional |
| 3. Posterior Fontanel | 7. Frontal Eye Fields | 12. Temporal Emotional |
| 4. Menopausal—Glandular (below and left of Posterior Fontanel) | 8. Fissure of Rolando | 13. Kidney |
| | 9. Parietal | |

## ZONE THERAPY

'When the nerves of the eyes and the feet are properly understood, there will be less need for surgical intervention,' said Dr Osler.

Most of us are familiar with the stories the spine can tell us, as every day we hear of the wonderful work of osteopaths, chiropractors and physiotherapists. A simple explanation of the results obtained in zone therapy, which is applied to the endocrine areas of the feet, is that the human body is an electro-mechanism. In this section I will give a detailed account of how to apply foot and sole zone therapy, for good results in relieving symptoms caused by abnormal glandular activity.

Many of us do not realise the importance of the tiny endocrine glands, but miraculous results can be achieved by applying a form of compression massage to the feet, in order to activate the reflex (located in the centre of each big toe) leading to the pituitary gland. Owing to the location of this important gland at the base of the brain, it should be remembered that any congestion in the back of the neck or its surrounding area will retard the blood supply and create a condition which would not exist if the circulation was not interfered with. Here lies the root cause of many nervous breakdowns. Fear, worry and sorrow causes an excessive build-up of toxins, which affects the chemical content of the blood and in turn increases nervous hypertension. Any treatment that relieves nervous tension sufficiently to create a renewed amount of circulation will eventually eliminate the toxins. I have already said that there is only one disease, physical or mental – congestion. If we relieve tension by removing congestion from the nerve extremities through the endocrine glands, good health will result.

I have taught the triune polarity of the body and its energies. With zone therapy, one will obtain miraculous effects if these polarities are accessed and utilised. It is the combined use of the head (cranial therapy), or positive pole, the feet (zone therapy), or negative pole, and the hands (zone therapy), or neutral pole, that allows the endocrines to have the most effect. This is an important statement; it has never before been considered in endocrine glandular balance, nor has this balance ever been used in the suggested fashion.

People should realise the importance of taking better care of their feet – neglect will generally lead to sickness. It must be realised that every corn, callous or bunion, depending on their location, will ultimately affect some organ or tissue of the body. Any undue pressure on the end of a nerve will have a definite effect on the organs involved. Make sure you keep your feet in good condition and visit a chiropodist regularly.

## HARMONY IN MIND AND BODY
Our bodies are wonderfully made. Harmony is necessary. Our body, mind and soul need rejuvenation.

'It's just a case of nerves' is a very common phrase, but in fact the human nervous system is the most highly developed communications system in the world, even more advanced than satellite communication or the most sophisticated computers. Of the millions of messages that pass through the central switchboard in the brain, only a fraction are under our control and these are related to what might be compared to outgoing calls. It is through having such control that we are able to walk, talk and eat.

It is the outgoing messages we *cannot* control that cause problems. Normally, when we eat the stomach releases digestive juices, because it is ordered to do so by the brain. The glands in the stomach release hydrochloric acid and the gastric glands provide pepsin. When we have an infection or an injury, white blood corpuscles (leukocytes) rush to the defence against infection. When invading bacteria or viruses are too powerful, the dead white blood corpuscles collect as pus and can cause an abscess if no ready outlet is found. At the first sign of oxygen deprivation, SOS messages are transmitted to the brain.

If there is stress in the body, however, when we eat little or no food, digestive juices are secreted and the first failure in protein digestion occurs. Such a deficiency creates additional stress, and the alarm signals continue until exhausted. Supplemental digestive enzymes would not only ensure better protein digestion, but would prevent nerve stress as well. When inborn metabolic errors exist and are unrecognised or not compensated for, susceptibility to any genetic weakness is increased.

What we see, hear, smell, taste or touch is instantly transmitted to the brain on the *incoming* line. Just like a telephone, we have no control over any incoming messages. To cope with the overload of incoming messages associated with modern living, the nervous system often needs extra nutrition, just as heavy physical work calls for extra food. Otherwise, the wires become overloaded and nervous exhaustion results.

When infective germs are encountered in daily living, the reserves of vitamins A and C, organic iron and calcium are not sufficient, and therefore an illness that could otherwise have been avoided 'catches' us. Trace elements and minerals are among the first line of defence of the nervous system. Normally present when nutrition is adequate, and digestion and assimilation satisfactory, these mighty midgets act as transmitters between the brain and the nerve network. When deficient, short-circuiting is common and often unrecognised. Primary among 'nerve foods' are the B vitamins, of which a continuing supply is needed, as well as the phosphate form of calcium, magnesium and sodium. Unrefined, biologically grown foods can supply such nutrients, but if we overlook food supplementation to ensure their presence, each meal is too much like Russian roulette for peace of mind.

Our mind and brain are two of the main things we have to keep in order. The one thing my mother prayed for all her life was that her brain cells would not deteriorate and her thoughts would remain clear. The brain is a marvellous organ and a great gift from our Creator, as Alfred Vogel always said. We would be lost without it; we could not plan, carry out or complete anything. So we have every reason to be grateful for it, every day of our lives. If a person voluntarily abstains from food or is made to go hungry and, as a result, loses a great deal of weight, the weight loss in the spinal cord and brain is hardly noticeable. The fact that everything else is affected first shows the importance of the brain as the control centre of every other process in the body.

Alfred Vogel made a comparison between the human brain and the walnut. The hard shell can be compared to the cranium. The two-lobed seed resembles the cerebrum, and the skin – which peels off easily in freshly picked nuts – may be likened to the meninges. At the back of the head, between the spinal cord and the brain, lies the cerebellum, which is approximately the size of an orange.

As Vogel so rightly said, the functions of the brain, as far as they have been discovered, are amazing. Picture, if you will, the control room of a large power plant or a modern ocean liner, or the instrument panels of a jet plane. All the numerous instruments and switches elicit our amazement and admiration. These control centres are, in a manner of speaking, the brain of the ship or plane. Everything that takes place, every change in direction, every response to the changeable elements, every command, comes from that control centre – the brain. The energy needed to make everything function is supplied by generators which produce energy, or power. When the power supply is insufficient or fails completely, it can be put down to problems in the central control, because it is either malfunctioning or out of action. This can happen even though engines and equipment have been designed and built in spectacular ways.

What can we learn from the above illustration? Alfred Vogel explains that energy is supplied to the brain via the bloodstream. If the blood carries all the necessary nutrients, nutritive salts and vitamins to ensure every brain cell receives the food it needs, everything will function properly. It is important to remember that the millions of cells do not each have separate functions: the brain is divided into work groups, called centres, and more than 20 of these centres have so far been recognised.

How an entire centre can be put out of order is seen in the case of a stroke. The attack usually occurs in the inner capsule and not the outer part of the brain, or cerebral cortex. If a blood vessel on the right side of the inner capsule ruptures, the blood supply to the outer parts of the brain is disrupted and the consequences appear on the left side of the body. This inversion is due to the fact that the cerebral hemisphere controls the opposite side of the body. Whatever we sense on the right side is registered on the left side and vice versa. If the body is able to repair the damage, the paralysis will pass and the ability to speak, which was lost, will return. If the speech centre remains disturbed, while the centre governing the connecting ideas continues to function, the person will be in the embarrassing position of thinking correctly but talking in a muddled way. However, this would not happen if that person were to write their thoughts instead of trying to express them verbally.

If we look at our body and all its functions, and at our mind and all its functions, where does it leave us? If we cut our body, blood flows, but if we 'cut' into our brain and our thoughts and emotions, the process is completely different – various emotions will be produced, such as aggression, a bad or unbalanced mood, or love. So, yes, the function of the mind is different.

It always astonishes me how the mind works. When I look at people who have held important managerial positions in their careers, who are very intelligent and run large companies, it seems devastating that they sometimes come to a time in life when they sit and play like children, or make no sense at all when speaking. When people are young, they never imagine anything will happen to them and, yet, because of senile dementia, or Alzheimer's, a total dysfunction of the mind, these normal, intelligent people can become like vegetables. In my student days, I often stayed with an aunt and uncle. My uncle had a managerial position in one of the largest psychiatric institutions in Holland. When I went there with him and he talked to the patients, I wondered how he could conduct conversations with people who could not be understood. At Christmas, we organised parties for even the most seriously affected patients, and their friendliness and love was obvious, but also the hate, anger and aggression that they felt.

I remember meeting a person there whom I admired for his writings (he had written many books) and the philosophies that he spread, who had ended up as a patient in that very hospital. I once had a chat with him. For the first five minutes we had an interesting conversation and I thought there was nothing wrong with him. However, after that very short period, his mind went completely and I had to be pulled away from him as a result of the aggressive attacks that he had. One wonders how the mind works. It shows us that the brain is just another organ and that the thoughts and emotions become reality by their interactions. As I have often said, the train gets to its destination only if every plug is in the right socket.

So much research has been done on the electrochemistry of the brain and how this can be corrected. Many scientists have also done their best to find out how the endocrine and immune systems really work. How is it possible that the endocrine system can be in such turmoil that a woman with premenstrual tension can actually murder the husband she so dearly loves? How is it possible to develop a Jekyll and Hyde personality? In my work in British prisons – with women as well as men – I have studied this phenomena over and over again. I have spoken to women in prisons who dearly loved their partners and yet committed a crime when their hormone systems were imbalanced, or male prisoners who, because of a totally wrong diet, became so aggressive that they committed murder. I have talked a great deal on this subject, even in the House of Lords, and have asked for understanding of British prisoners and their diet, for nutrition and mental behaviour are often the cause of unnecessary crimes and the wrong mental behaviour. We sometimes dismiss the brain, but it operates on the same biochemical principles as any other part of the anatomy.

It is said that over 40,000 people commit suicide in Europe each year. Depression – especially clinical depression – is still very much misunderstood. The mind, body and soul, which work together, are often treated separately but should really be considered as one unit. Drugs are not always the answer; they are often not the whole story in balancing the body. A holistic approach to the problems associated with depression, mood swings and mental behaviour would work better. I have tried to explain in the first part of this book that the body works as an electrical field, and electrical and magnetic therapies can be of help. 'Cure' is a very big word. Before we can begin to find all the answers to this very complex subject, we have to learn a lot more about the body as a whole, and its hormonal balances.

I remember when Roger MacDougall and I went to a university to try to convince a professor there of the benefits of a gluten-free diet. We told him that we were of the opinion that gluten, which has an influence on bowel tissue, can also have an influence on brain tissue. We mentioned that we had seen some promising results with schizophrenia, and also with autism and autistic children, with a gluten-free diet. That was about 20 years ago, when we were dismissed as two nutcases who did not know what they were talking about. Many universities have now proved that gluten-free diets are often very successful in treating an autistic child. It is wonderful to see what can be done by simply adjusting the diet.

For 45 years, I have worked with St John's wort (*Hypericum perforatum*), as a fresh extract, since Alfred Vogel and I researched it many years ago and realised what a wonderful remedy it is. By its characteristics and signatures, we can see the purpose it was created for. If we take a leaf and put it under a microscope, we can see it is covered with tiny little holes, filled with healing oil. It has many beneficial properties, even in the cosmetic acupuncture work I do on scars and blemishes. St John's wort is named after the apostle of love and, as a herb, it says to us, 'I love you, I want to heal you.' It is beneficial for blood circulatory problems and also as a remedy to heal the mind. Lots of research has been carried out on St John's wort and there has also been a lot of criticism of it, but it is a wonderful remedy if properly prescribed.

We now know that omega-3, essential fatty acids, are not only good for the heart but also for the brain. We see this with hyperactive and autistic children. Again, every case has to be treated individually and personally diagnosed. We see this so often with problems associated with mental behaviour. Nutrition, as I have written in my book, *Viruses, Allergies and the Immune System*, is essential. What kind of remedies can one prescribe for so many of these systemic disorders? We often see how emotional a patient can be who has heart problems, or how depressed a cancer patient can be. If a negative mood can swing to become positive, then medicines could be successful in helping with these different forms of depressions and nervous anxiety.

So many treatments are aimed at restoring electrochemical imbalances alone but, again, I see the body as a whole. It is so much better to treat mental problems in that way. Stress can often be controlled by simple methods such as breathing exercises, acupuncture, meditation and remedies to balance the hormonal system. In several of my books, I have written about the endocrines and how much the pineal gland, and other glands we know very little about, are subjected to control that lies within our reach. If one of the endocrines is out of balance, they all are. It is therefore important that the output, or release, of hormonal substances, controlled by the endocrine system, is balanced; the responsibility to lead a more sensible life lies within ourselves. In modern society, where the world is hurried and stress is an 'in' word, we have to realise that we might have to make adjustments to our lifestyles in order to set aside a little more time for ourselves. We have only scratched the surface of what we can do with these conditions, and much more research and understanding is needed.

Nature is our best friend and we can learn a lot from nature, and what is given to assist us, like St John's wort and gingko biloba. If we examine the gingko leaf, it is astonishing how much it looks like the brain and, again, it tells us with its characteristics and signatures that we should use it for help in this area. The gingko tree is commonly called the 'memory tree'. If we look at the leaf, we see that it is very heavy and made of two halves, held together by a very little stem. It is a wonder of nature that this leaf not only helps improve memory but also aids circulation and conditions that often affect the mind.

More clinical trials are necessary to establish the value and efficacy of these herbs. Sometimes we may observe in amazement how effectively certain remedies work, but research is needed to look at their healing properties in more depth. There is so much out there in nature to help us. A tremendous amount of money has been spent on discovering more about the moon, but resources must also be provided to research our own flora and fauna, in order to find possible cures for many illnesses.

We often look to the scientific world for help, but we have to accept its failings. We have simple phrases, like 'you are what you eat', but we haven't really fully researched what a low-stress diet can do to relieve tensions in the body. I discovered this with one of the prisoners I treated. He had five allergies and is now a completely different person, simply through making some dietary adjustments. He was lost in a world where his only help was a gun to quieten his mind and he often said that the only pleasure he had in life was murder. After I discovered the allergies which were affecting his life so drastically and treated him by cutting out certain foods and desensitising him, he became a different person and was liked by people. He is now trying to make up for all the bad things he has done. It was interesting that when Princess Anne visited him, he told her the story of how his life had changed since his allergies were treated and the alteration this had made to his brain. I still see him regularly and when I look at him and remember what he was once like, I realise the amazing difference nutrition can make.

It is true that we are what we eat and drink. It is a good idea not only to look at foods that might mop up free radicals or cleanse the body, but also to investigate foods that will help change our mood. In the many books I have written on the hidden dangers in food and drink and nature's gift of food, I have shown how much we can support our mind by cutting out stress-related foods like caffeine, alcohol, chocolate, nicotine, sugar and salt – all things that will influence our stress levels. Ways of changing from a high-stress diet to a low-stress one are explained in detail in a few of these books. The link between food and mental behaviour is not a new thing. Even in the nineteenth century people wrote about it. However, more research is needed to find out exactly what that relationship is and also to explain anti-social behaviour.

There are so many things that can help. When I look at some of the patients I have treated, it is a comfort to know that one does not need to live with a problem, but can overcome it with a realistic, sensible approach. Our mind and body can be in harmony again, and unwanted mental conditions can be beaten.

A typical case comes to mind. One evening, I was called by a medical consultant to see his son. He was a very promising young boy with his future mapped out, a bright student with a brilliant brain. Towards the end of his university career, he got involved in a relationship. When this relationship broke down he began to feel suicidal. He battled with the problem and his work suffered. As he had previously had glandular fever, his immune system deteriorated rapidly and he became very vulnerable to illness. The poor fellow became very tired and ill, and developed ME (also known as Post-viral Fatigue Syndrome). In medical circles, ME is often misunderstood and he had a tough battle on his hands to get his problems recognised. A lot of time and money was spent trying to help this young man, but he eventually became so ill that he had to lie in a darkened room and could not stand any daylight. He battled on and many times I sat with him in this dark room, completely away from light, with the windows blackened out. One evening during one of our many talks, he became quite aggressive and violent, but I kept trying to reassure him that things would work out in time. Very slowly, after an extremely long time, he began to pick up, realised that life was worth living and slowly recovered. At that time, his mind was stronger than his body. Positively, he tried with the help of some audio tapes and wonderful remedies to get better.

The very first thing for people suffering from such conditions, especially when they have, or have had, glandular fever is to carry out detoxification. Supplementation with *Daily Choice of Antioxidants* was essential in the case of this young man. Following a blood test, I also used strong remedies to dissipate strong poisonous materials in his system. He reacted very well to *Centaurium* from Bioforce which can give brilliant results in such cases, and *Eleutherococcus*, to give him a boost. Each morning, he drank a glass of beetroot juice to rid his body of toxic materials and slowly but surely, especially after liver cleansing with *Milk Thistle Complex*, he recovered. He is a happy young man again and can now look forward to a bright future, despite his terrible experience.

Too often with ME the mind can become extremely involved and, because of the excessive tiredness associated with the illness, if corrective measures are not taken things can be disastrous.

Despite having treated this condition for so many years, I was really shocked when a young woman came to see me one Saturday morning accompanied by her husband. I could see that her condition was very advanced and that she really needed help. I told her husband that he should take extra care of her and that she needed a lot of rest, and advised him what to do. At the time, she was very grateful to get help but a few days later something disastrous happened. I later learned that whilst out in the car with her husband and children, she drove straight into a river and the whole family drowned. Such cases shake one even after many years in practice. One can try to help and do the very best to help with human suffering, but when a patient's mental state gets as bad as that, things become very difficult.

Another case that comes to my mind is that of a minister who was totally addicted to sodium amytal. I was shocked to learn that he sometimes took 30 or even 40 tablets of this substance when he had to conduct a service. I spoke to him and asked how he could promise his parishioners eternal life when he was basically killing himself. I told him that I could only speak to him through sodium amytal and could not get through to him as a person, because he was completely drugged. He was a bit shocked when I told him that the mind is stronger than flesh and bones, and asked why we should bother if we believe that the spirit stays alive. In the next part of this book, we will discuss this further. I talked many times to this minister and slowly, with the help of acupuncture, *avena sativa*, *Neuroforce* and some stronger remedies like *Enhanced Nerve Factor*, I slowly managed to get him off the drug. When he came to grips with life again, he found that there was much more to it than sodium amytal.

You must first recognise the problem and then decide what steps must be taken in order to help. Talking about this, I am reminded of a particular lady whom I have treated now for many years. When she initially came to see me she was very irrational and nervous, and had developed a condition that appeared to be like schizophrenia. She told me in great detail that she believed there were spirits around her, chasing her and making her life miserable, and indeed pestering the life out of her continually. I could not understand this case because she still managed to run a business. In her job, she seemed so normal that no one would have realised there was anything wrong with her. Her husband, a very nice man, told me that psychiatrists were actually mystified as, although she was thought to be schizophrenic, she didn't have all the symptoms of this disorder. I talked over the whole problem with her and we came to several conclusions in relation to her great unhappiness. She had no fulfilment generally and had slowly developed this condition, as she described it, 'with evil spirits ruling her life'. I decided to talk to her about a gluten- and sugar-free diet and based the treatment on a few things she told me about her food intake. To cut a long story short, she managed to improve and could cope more easily with the responsibilities she had in life. She was helped by several remedies, such as zinc, and *Health Insurance Plus*, a vitamin, which made sure that she would not develop deficiencies because of the adjustments we made to her diet. She also took some homoeopathic remedies. She responded well and the 'evil spirits', as she called them, slowly vanished. As I have said, the mind is stronger than the body, but it is still necessary to recognise aspects of nutrition that may be causing problems.

Something that happened not very long ago reminded me how important dietary management is. As a gluten-free diet is very helpful for MS patients, it is now well recognised that it is also useful in treating autistic children. There have been some reports from universities claiming that gluten can have an influence on health, and I especially feel that omitting gluten and sugar from the diet is very good for certain conditions. I treated one particular young boy for a long time, until I could get no further. It was not until I finally persuaded his parents to put him on a gluten-free diet that he improved. What a great delight it was when he spoke for the first time, picking up my telephone and saying, 'Hello Daddy'. The parents were absolutely delighted and that helped them put their faith in helping him normalise himself through diet.

Another patient comes to my mind, who went through a very difficult experience. She settled here after coming from another country. She had difficulties finding work and finally got a job working for an elderly couple. She devoted her life to this couple and treated them as she would have wished to be treated herself. However, the pressures were high. Unfortunately, the couple died within six weeks. Their deaths made it very difficult for her and put her under tremendous strain. She developed a nasty candida and then, much worse, a brain tumour was diagnosed. Unfortunately, this was so serious that she needed an operation. Following the operation, which left her slightly handicapped, she came to see me. She had not eradicated her candida because she had not been keeping strictly to her diet. After encouraging her to cooperate, I told her doctors that it was not the after-effect of the brain tumour that needed treatment, but the candida. Luckily they agreed. I got a personal letter from them saying that the girl undoubtedly got much better after her candida had been treated.

It takes a lot of understanding to discover the offenders in any illness. Once again, physical, mental and emotional balance is necessary to overcome many health problems. One lady I treated suffered from very bad insomnia. She could not get to sleep, and became nervous and extremely anxious. I asked her to read my book, *Stress and Nervous Disorders*, which was a great help to her. I also advised her to read *Inner Harmony*. After having acupuncture and taking natural remedies for sleep, she improved greatly – she became more motivated and realised that life had more to offer her than living with this fear that she could not sleep. She had developed a fear of fear, which always exacerbates the condition. Again, her mind became stronger and more positive after I taught her a few simple methods she could practice at home, and she improved so much that she has now resumed a normal life.

Recently I got a letter that was simply signed 'A Mum'. The letter was about her son, who saw me a few times. In it she reveals that he was a lovely son, but had become very strange. He had a few disappointments with girlfriends and, while he was growing up, there were a lot of problems as he did not get on well with his father. He became unhappy. He spent a lot of time alone in his room and, one day, his mother discovered that he had started to dress himself up as a girl. He also developed some nasty behavioural problems, which made life very difficult for his mother. In addition to this, he stole money from her to buy clothes to dress up in and other odd habits surfaced. Suddenly he developed strange sexual behaviour. He then started to steal women's clothing from other people. This lady wrote to me saying she was going out of her mind and did not know who to turn to. Nobody would believe her because he seemed such a nice, caring boy and everyone thought she must feel very proud of him. She felt very alone having to cope with this situation and asked for my help. Cases like this need a lot of care and monitoring, in addition to good guidance. I advised her to take certain steps to help her son and how she could find suitable people to counsel him. I also helped her as I felt very sorry for her. Seeing what a state the poor boy was in, I also tried to motivate him in a different direction.

Often, addictions of the mind can really affect people – not only gambling, alcohol and nicotine, but all kinds of addictions. Self-will has to be used and self-control must be exercised. In my book, *Inner Harmony*, I give several ways to treat these conditions and balance the physical, mental and emotional bodies.

One Saturday morning, a delightful couple came to see me. He was a very hard-working businessman who was under terrific pressure. I had already given him a lot of help with his arthritis, but he got very worked up and nervous because of the tremendous financial strain he was under, being the director of a money-lending business. She was an equally nice person, but was always ill. We had some good talks together. He found the acupuncture very helpful for relaxation, but often found that, although he had a lovely wife, she was a drain on him because she never seemed to get any better. Even before she sat down in the chair in my consulting room, she told me that she never felt well – she was always nervous and fed up, did not sleep well and could not socialise with other people. She had no willpower to get better. On this particular Saturday morning, she was again anxious to tell me how bad she felt. I sat her down in the presence of her husband. I felt very sorry for her, but I had to do it, and began telling her a few home truths. I said she would never get any better as she was so anxious to tell the world how ill she was, and there was no way at all that her situation would improve unless she took some positive action in her life. I asked her bluntly, 'Why are you always ill?' Physically, she had nothing wrong with her. As her husband sat in silence, I gave her such a talking to that I felt she would never come back to see me. Then I told her that we would try acupuncture and other treatments, but that I was sorry, I could not help her any further if she did not change her attitude. I gave her a few examples of what other people who had similar problems and took themselves in hand did to get better. The key to her own recovery was in her own hands. She had to do it herself. She left my consulting room feeling down, but to my surprise they both came back two weeks later. Indeed, she was very much better and her husband said to me, very quietly, 'The last treatment was really the best.' From then on, I offered her encouragement and saw her blossoming. Although I always found her a very nice person, she actually became much more attractive and pleasant and gave them both a new lease of life. I met them at the airport years later, looking very happy. He had retired and she supported him in every way, and had a much happier attitude to life.

As I have so often said, the mind is stronger than the body. It will direct the body, not the other way around, and therefore it is very helpful to sit down sometimes and talk to oneself and make sure that whatever treatment (orthodox or alternative) you receive, you are positive and have the desire to make it work. In the next part of this book, I will describe a great friend to encourage us with physical and mental problems.

# SOUL

Try to imagine a very close friend who is extremely clever and who you can speak to on a wide range of subjects. Suddenly, out of the blue, they plead, 'You have to help me because I feel soulless. I have little spirituality and you need to tell me what to do to correct this.' This happened to me, with a friend. As we can usually talk together on an intelligent level, I asked her what she knew about the soul. She told me that having been brought up in a strict religious environment, she understood a little, but always had the desire to be more spiritual. I know of no one who does more good work than her. She is always helping others, especially the less privileged. She makes every effort to support them as much as she possibly can where there is a need. However, it does not necessarily follow that living a good life and caring about the well-being of others means that one is good to oneself, nourishing the soul.

I discussed this subject many times with Alfred Vogel and would like to pass on a few of the thoughts on which we agreed. Over the years I have learned a lot about the importance of nourishing the soul. Our spirituality depends a lot on how much time and effort we put into our own soul, which has been entrusted to us from birth.

I saw this clearly when one of my grandchildren, Gemma, was born, weighing only 1 lb 8 oz. Very few people thought she would survive. However, that tiny baby had a great will to live and with the small amount of life that was in her little body, she did everything she could to fight against all the monitors and drains that were being used to keep her alive. When it was said that she would not survive, I disagreed. I knew that everything would turn out well, because I could see that her breathing was in perfect harmony and that God had given her the breath of life, which is valuable to all of us. She is a very blessed child who, at

127

the young age of six, has a spirituality that shines from within her.

In receiving the breath of life, the soul that God gives us to help us become his children, we go a little bit higher than being merely the children of man. God created the first man with a living soul in his own image and likeness. That is why it is often said that we should be the image of God, himself imperfect, but perfect in the eyes of his own son, Christ. When God 'formed man of the dust of the ground [one might even say of the elements of the earth] and breathed into his nostrils the breath of life, man became a living soul' (Genesis 2, verse 7), a living creature. It is also said that God poured out his soul into this creature. When we think about these particular passages in the Good Book, we see that humankind represents emotion in life, in all its complexity.

The environment we grow up in has an influence on the soul. A revealing story comes to mind that a very good friend of mine, who actually knew the people involved, told me. A family who lived on the border of a forest suddenly got an enormous shock when their young baby, who was outside in the back garden in a pram, disappeared. They were devastated and searched the entire area, but the baby had vanished. Naturally, it was assumed that the baby had been stolen and would never be seen again. Obviously the family was in total despair. One day, many years later, the local blacksmith watched a group of gorillas. As he had been brought up in the country and understood animal behaviour very well, he noticed that one of them was acting strangely. He later returned to the gorillas with some other people who were more knowledgeable, and they watched it. They realised that somehow they had to entice this gorilla away from the others so that further investigations could be carried out. After their investigations, they realised that the 'gorilla' was actually a human being, with an altogether different life than the rest. After checking its DNA, they concluded that this was in fact the baby who had been stolen all those years ago. It was surmised that one of the gorillas had lifted the baby from the pram, brought it into their community, fed the baby and brought it up as one of their own. Although it was very scared, it was not as frightened of humans as the rest of the gorillas, and this was what had initially alerted the man. The human soul of the baby showed a disparity between animal and man. It was then that my friend, who studied problems relating to the soul, saw how much the environment influenced behaviour, and it reminded him that we have a soul that is totally different from the soul of an animal.

God created a lifeless body, a conglomeration of cells, and then He charged that body with the breath of life. The spirits began to permeate the lifeless form and then, when life entered it, and man became conscious of himself, he began to breathe and became a living soul. This made us complete beings, with physical, mental and emotional bodies, for as I have said many times, we are not one body, but three. The breath of life is the living soul, and must be considered as a whole.

We often find that a negative reaction takes place in the physical and emotional body when there is mental disturbance. It is well known that physical afflictions leave their mark on the patient and, in turn, impose further restrictions upon the body. This field still has to be explored further as we do not know much about the hormonal system or, for instance, the pineal gland, which is an aerial to the cosmos and is instrumental in harmonising the body with the rest of Creation.

I told the dear friend who asked me to help her overcome her spiritual problems that the first thing she had to do was sit down and meditate, learn to understand herself better, have a good inward look at herself and then carry out my specially designed breathing exercises. As I have said, the breath of life is essential.

A little story I told her also helped. While I was in China, there was a young, hard-working surgeon whom I admired for her tremendous energy. When I asked what she did to relax, she told me that her parents and grandparents had taught her a breathing exercise called hara breathing. This particular breathing involves breathing slowly and rhythmically through the nose, deep into the stomach and out through the mouth. I asked my friend to sit down, to meditate and then put her left hand on the tummy (about half an inch under the navel) and place the right hand over the left hand. At that point, a magnetic ring on the vital centre of the body – the hara – is formed. The Chinese have an old saying that the navel is the gateway to everything. It is also the last part of a baby's body to become divorced from its mother. Here is an interesting fact: if you put the left hand on the navel and the right hand on top, leaving your legs uncrossed, no hypnotist will ever be able to get through to you, because you have formed a magnetic ring that brings you into perfect harmony with yourself and with Creation. To continue the hara breathing exercise, breathe slowly in through the nose, filling your mouth with air, while keeping your ribcage still. Don't breathe into your breast, but deep down into your tummy and out through your mouth, very gently and slowly, in and out, as if you are walking in a garden and smelling a lovely flower. Concentrate your mind on your stomach and breathe in slowly. Once your stomach is filled with air, round the lips and slowly breathe out, pulling in the muscles to flatten your stomach. This can be done as often as desired. The sensation after finishing is normally either one of complete relaxation and a desire for sleep, or of refreshment and the desire to return to work. This exercise sounds easier than it is, but it actually takes a little time to master properly. I cannot over-emphasise the importance of breathing properly.

When children start to grow and develop their own personalities their breathing pattern changes. A relaxed child will breathe into the stomach, giving the vegetative nervous system a real treat. With correct breathing, the soul also gets nourishment, which is extremely important. Without this, we know that when the soul starves, the body starves and consequently this contributes further to a lack of spirituality. It is therefore very important to get the breathing right.

I remarked to my worried friend that she must have studied the energy of light, and I feel that light is the future of medicine. Because she had a religious upbringing and believed in Creation, when I asked her what the first thing God created was, she immediately said, 'Light, because the Book tells us that God said "Let there be light and there was light."' Then I asked her, 'How do you think this is possible? On the fourth day, God created the sun, the moon and the stars, so how could there have been light beforehand?' This puzzled her and she looked at me as if to find an answer. I told her how important it was that she fed her soul and gained spirituality because that was exactly what God did – on the first day he created a spiritual light – and we can read further about this in the bible in Second Corinthians (chapter 4, verse 6), when Paul said, 'For God, who commanded the light to shine out of darkness, hath shined in our hearts, to give the light of the knowledge of the glory of God in the face of Jesus Christ.' That is the reason we read in St John's epistle that Jesus's life was the light of human life, and this makes us children of light (chapter 12, verse 36), producing all the wonderful characteristics that my dear friend was aiming for.

This is frequently misunderstood, but once we have

discovered that special light, we can do all things through Christ, who gives us the power. It is quite amazing to experience how powerful we can then become when we accept that particular spiritual light, which is even more important than the natural light that appeared when God created the sun, the moon and the stars. Possessing spirituality makes us better people and I strongly believe that the future of medicine is to gain more knowledge about the spiritual light that is the real nourishment for the soul.

When imbalanced people start to learn and understand a little bit more about this topic they often improve, and when they undergo treatment of the imbalances light is very good as it is also attuned to colour. In his wonderful book, *Living Proof: A Medical Mutiny*, Prof. Michael Gearing-Tosh, who shows how he beat cancer, puts strong emphasis on the breathing exercises that I taught him and, through those exercises, became determined to do more to help himself.

## COLOUR THERAPY

Isaac Newton would have been amazed to know how much he has done for medicine with his discovery of gravity. In 1666, Newton also discovered that sunlight did not consist of a single golden-white colour, as was believed until then, but was made up of indigo, violet, blue, green, yellow, orange and red. His breakthrough led other scientists to wonder which of these colours or groups of colours in the spectrum were responsible for the curative powers of the sun. The word spectrum, derived from a Latin word meaning 'image', is employed to indicate measured wavelengths given off by rays such as the visible coloured rays of the sun, and the invisible rays found above and below the coloured rays, as revealed by the spectroscope. This is an instrument containing an optical prism, which breaks a beam of light up into the visible colours of the spectrum and disperses these colours on to a reflecting surface. When the spiritual light within us is exercised by prayer, meditation and being in tune with nature, the physical and mental body will improve if we introduce light and colour therapy.

In the year 1800, Sir William Herschel discovered that there was an area lower in the spectrum than the lowest visible colour (red) which caused a thermal meter to register an even higher degree of heat than that of the red area. The following year, Johann Ritter discovered there were rays above those of the visible violet ray found at the top of the spectrum. These rays were called ultraviolet rays, 'ultra' being derived from the Latin word meaning 'beyond', and the discoveries of both infrared and ultraviolet rays have since played an extremely important part in light therapy.

The gradual steps of scientific enquiry gave us first of all sunlight alone, as a means of applying light therapy (or heliotherapy), then by studying the rays of the sun, the colours of the spectrum were discovered.

The theory of light therapy is well established and the wavelengths of the rays determine which type of treatment will be given. Most of the longer rays (including some of the visible rays) heat the blood and accelerate all kinds of colour therapy, stimulate circulation and assist in pain relief. Through wearing certain colours hormonal balance can very often be achieved, as I have described in my books, *Menstrual and Premenstrual Tension* and *Menopause*.

I talked to my friend about all this for a considerable time and she became very interested. She is always keen to broaden her knowledge, and understood my explanation of Creation and light. She felt very well physically and mentally, and well balanced. I told her the endocrine system played an important part in this, especially for women but also, to some extent, for men.

There is a spiritual system as well as a physical one. As I have said, the pineal gland (which is the aerial to the cosmos) sends messages to the other glands and they have to work in harmony. In other words, the seven chakras, which are the centres of the life force, need to be fed. I still believe that an undernourished soul influences this life force and can lead not only to hormonal imbalance, but also to disease. Unity in the body needs to be looked at from every angle and I have often seen the benefits gained. I feel that spiritual and natural light are extremely necessary, and light and colour therapy are important. This form of therapy is not a gimmick and, as I told my friend, in the words of Shakespeare: 'There are more things in heaven and earth . . . than are dreamt of in your philosophy.'

It is interesting to look at the advances that have been made in this field. The late Parsee scientific genius, Dr Dinshah P. Ghadiali, has made a tremendous contribution to medicine with his studies of colour and light. He invented a special machine called a spectrochrometer, in which the colour lenses are so perfectly aligned and attuned that they synchronise exactly with the speed and frequency of the vibrations of the different colours of light visible on this planet. He also established how the essences of the different elements of the mineral kingdom of earth come from our solar system through sunbeams and how each element, when analysed through this instrument, reveals through the prism of reflected colours of light a tendency towards a particular colour. He scientifically showed the effect each colour has on the organs and other parts of the body and which colour should be used for the treatment of various diseases. This has benefited me greatly over the years when deciding on the correct treatment for patients. I have been able to use colour therapy in combination with other treatments, and have had especially good results when combining it with acupuncture. As a result of this, many patients with nervous breakdowns or even suicidal tendencies have experienced great improvement and relief.

My dear friend, Prof. Meher K. Master, often supports the wonderful work of Dr Ghadiali in her seminars. Until fairly recently laser-beam light therapy was practically unknown, but today we have some awareness of the tremendous power of light. The wonderful invention of this particular machine deserves worldwide recognition for the tremendous relief it has given people.

The endocrine system especially is very susceptible to colour therapy. Our knowledge of this system is still insufficient – not even endocrinologists could give us a full explanation of how it works – but we do know that this system is greatly affected by colour and light. Sometimes I remind people that there are:

- seven endocrine glands
- seven layers in the solar spectrum
- seven layers of light receptors in the eye retina
- seven basic scale steps in the musical octave

In one of my books, *Cancer and Leukaemia*, I gave several examples of how colour affects these glands and, indeed, how it affects our whole life. I have seen:

- the pineal gland react to violet
- the pituitary gland to cyanogen blue
- the thyroid gland to green
- the thymus to yellow

- the pancreas to orange
- the adrenals to orange-red, and
- the gonads to red

To find harmony in this octave, it is important to remember that the eyes, which are the ultimate example of all this, react very well to greenish-blue.

Over a long period, I have practised iridology in my clinics and it is most interesting when working with colour therapy to compare reactions before and after treatment. It is also beneficial to combine colour therapy with Kirlian photography, which is used to show the energy field, or aura, around the body. It makes a tremendous difference to patients and even boosts the immune system.

Just as there are seven divisions on the physical plane and seven colours in the rainbow, the energy known as 'sound' has seven musical notes in the scale and the first note recurs on the eighth key, at a higher or lower pitch depending on which side of the scale it appears. Dr Ghadiali, after years of thorough experiments and research, found that red, yellow and blue colours are not the fundamental colours of light. He established that the true triad of primary colours of light was red, green and violet, and the triad of secondary colours was yellow, blue and magenta. He formulated his method of treatment on the 12 colours of vibrant light. Red, orange, yellow, lemon, green, turquoise, blue, indigo, violet and the hidden or higher spiritual portion of the rainbow: purple, magenta and scarlet. It seems that magenta is the most significant colour frequency for evolution. In Ghadiali's writings, he mentions that just as the musical scale has seven main tones and five semi-tones, making a total of twelve, for instance on the piano keyboard seven white keys and five black keys, so too the spectrum of light is divided into seven main colours and five semi-tone colours, making a total of twelve. Each colour vibrates and oscillates at its own distinctive speed of wave formation. The power of light-colour formations and the change of the atomic weight of the element is the key to the transmutation of the so-called elements from one to another.

I remember a multiple sclerosis patient who did not show any progress when given acupuncture. When a very good friend of mine, who is also one of the best homoeopathic doctors I know, visited our clinic and suggested combining colour therapy with her ongoing treatment, the difference was incredible. Another patient, a diabetic aged about 65, suffered complications in her blood circulation as well as heart problems and was greatly discouraged. Yet, within three months of receiving gentle colour radiation treatment, she showed remarkable improvement.

Even with a homoeopathic approach, colour therapy is of tremendous help when combined with gem therapy. Gemstone treatment, as part of complete colour therapy, is very beneficial and the radiance of light serves as further evidence of the divine laws of nature. After all, it is said, 'From light we came, to light we return.'

Colour is the most valued gift of nature. What would it be like if we could only see things in black and white? Yet scientists have failed to analyse the recent advances in colour healing. Even in ancient times, colour was greatly appreciated, valued and understood, and in many parts of the world, particularly in Greece and Egypt, we know that there were temples dedicated to the worship of light and colour, especially the sun. It is with great thanks that we realise the power of colour in our lives. Scientifically, colour is a rate of vibration. The eye adjusts to let in certain amounts of light and the nerve endings at the back of the retina are sensitive to colour vibrations. To this end, harmony is necessary.

At one time in the United States of America, several children from one classroom suffered leukaemia. Finally, a colour specialist was called in, who suggested that their endocrine systems had reacted to an ill-matched range of colours in the room. When these colours were adjusted, the leukaemia incidence returned to normal. There is tremendous power in colour repulsions and affinities, which is really beyond human understanding. We only need to look at the seven different colours in sunlight and how each is composed of a different style and number of vibrations. Each colour has specific properties. The two unseen colours in the rainbow have an even greater meaning and can be used harmoniously in different therapies to the benefit of patients.

Nature's greatest gift of all is light and there are many publications on the use and value of infrared or ultraviolet light. However, very little has been written about the visible colour range of the spectrum. The primitive races saluted the rising and setting of the sun. Apart from everything else, without light there can be no life. Colour belongs to light, and colour is life; life is colour. How many things lose their efficacy when their colour is faded or lost? It is sometimes said that all energy is vibration and all vibration is energy. The vibrations of colour can produce great results with work in the human energy field. When harmonising colours are used at the right time, colour therapy can produce seemingly inexplicable results.

With the above in mind, I quote Albert Einstein:

> It is possible that there exist emanations that are still unknown to us. Do you remember how electrical current and 'unseen waves' were laughed at? The knowledge about man is still in its infancy.

In several of our clinics, we have a specialised, computerised treatment which, for many people, has been a great success.

My friend was very satisfied with our conversation and I am sure that she benefits from these little talks. Life is so wonderful and if we can see it in its reality, so much can be done to help ourselves improve matters where necessary.

A middle-aged lady comes to mind. She was very religious and had a lot of unanswered questions. As I told her, I don't have all the answers. I have struggled a lot with my own queries and have thought and prayed about them. But as I have said, as long as I make sure that the basics are right, I will get there. This lady felt she could do more in life, but had many doubts and wished life could just be the way she wanted it to be. She put a strange question to me when she asked, 'Who are we really and what place do we fill in life?' She said that she frequently looked into the past and had rejected the present. She often thought that she should be doing more worthwhile things in her life. I told her that in Exodus (chapter 3, verse 14) God said, 'I am.' When you dwell in the past, thinking of all the mistakes you have made and the regrets that you have, then you live alone. God said, 'I am that I am'; He did not say 'I was.' One has to look forward. Furthermore, if you live in the future with your problems and fears, you also live alone. 'I am not there, my name is not "I will be".' However, if you live in the present with faith in your heart, then you are not alone. 'I am always with you, my name is "I Am".' That is a great comfort, because we know that we can be helped by understanding more about the purpose of the soul, and also the purpose of life.

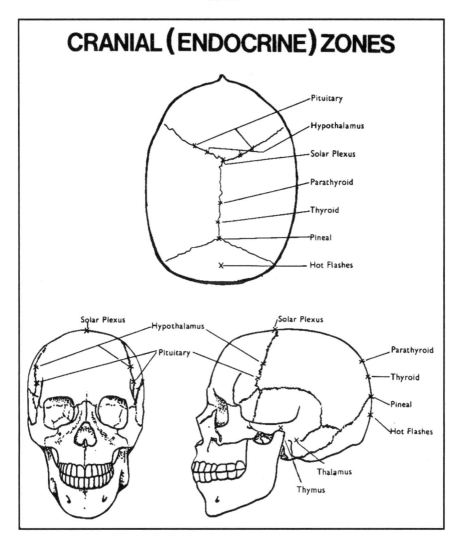

# CRANIAL (ENDOCRINE) ZONES

This reminds me of another patient who was very keen to become a better person. She wanted me to give her an illustration of what I really felt we should be. That is always very difficult, because one knows one's own soul better than anyone else. If we want to understand more about life, we should look to our Creator, who created everything in perfection. However, I passed on a story one of my very best friends told me, that I enjoyed immensely. It is about a silversmith. In the last book of the Old Testament it is said that God will 'sit as a refiner and purifier of silver' (Malachi, chapter 3, verse 3). Although this puzzled her a little bit, she found the image of the silversmith holding a piece of silver over the fire to heat interesting to envisage. The silversmith holds the silver in the middle of the fire, where the flames are the hottest, in order to burn away all the impurities, just as God holds us in a 'hot spot' to refine and purify us. The smith not only holds the silver, but also keeps an eye on it the entire time it is over the fire. If the silver was left for a moment too long in the flames, it would be destroyed. The final question, which is quite intriguing, is how it is possible to know when the silver is fully refined. The silversmith answers that easily: it is totally refined when he can see his image in it. When feeling the heat of the fire, we have to remember that God has his eye on us and will keep watching until He sees his image in us. That is a wonderful thought, as life can be difficult sometimes, but in order to become a better person in this world, you have to be able to cope with bad experiences too. It often baffles our human mind to see how Creation works and how we are looked after, for often our lives are saved from disasters beyond our own control.

Every day, we are surprised by our body chemistry. Life is full of emotion and, so often, taking positive action can solve problems. Negativity and positivity are two very important attitudes in life – positive will always win over negative. Negative emotions are related to body chemistry and this is widely recognised today, even in direct relation to degenerative diseases including cancer. The late Ernest Holmes, founder of the Science of Mind Institute, taught that resentment and self-pity are often related to the development of cancer; that the inability to forgive engenders stiff joints; that pleasing others in order to gain favour (in other words, being 'sweet') invites diabetes; and that anger, often hidden or suppressed, can be the unsuspected cause of high blood pressure, leading to strokes. The Chinese have long taught that the liver is an organ subject to emotional stress. Modern research offers realistic explanations of the phenomena involved. For instance, anger profoundly alters all organic apparatus, as the late Dr Alexis Carrell stated. In anger, muscles contract, the sympathetic nervous system and the suprarenal glands go into action, blood pressure increases, the heart races and the liver releases stored glucose into the blood, which is grabbed by the muscles as fuel. Circulation, respiration, digestion and the muscular-nerve apparatus are forced to act. Response to all stresses sets in high gear all body activities and adaptive functions. The hypothalamus, as part of the limbic system, has dominion over emotional expression and is responsible for the reaction pattern characteristic of rage. Conversely, a lazy hypothalamus may be responsible for the inability to fall in love! The hypothalamus also regulates homeostasis, including regulation of temperature, water balance, hypophysial (pituitary) function and gastric secretion, among other things. Hormone secretion through nervous input depends upon releasing and inhibiting factors originating in the hypothalamus, acting upon the hypophysis. The apostat, or satiety centre, is also located in the hypothalamus.

Like a chain reaction, when any one of the endocrine glands is over- or under-stimulated, a ripple or domino effect undulates through the system, first of all affecting areas of genetic weakness and those where circulation is inhibited. Nutritional deficiencies compound the stress. Fear, anger and depression can inhibit the secretion of hydrochloric acid, resulting in over-alkalinity, the breakdown or hydrolysis of proteins to amino acids, protein deficiency (even though the diet is adequate) and inevitable toxicity, or auto- (self-) toxication at cellular level. When anger or other negative emotions occur, separating the act from the actor helps to avoid inviting self-pity or resentment. Fortunate are those who communicate their feelings in an attitude of resolving differences, or meeting halfway for a fair compromise.

Emotions are usually learned, and take four major aspects:

1. recognition of a situation
2. expressing or giving external signs
3. experience of evaluation
4. excitement or intensity of the emotion

This reminds me of a businessman who told me that because of the disasters in his life (for instance, when his wife left him because his business failed) he had lost all faith. He had suffered a nervous breakdown and one of the awful things that happened to him was that he could no longer concentrate. It is often the case after an emotional disaster that one cannot concentrate or loses one's faith, as the soul is not receiving the nourishment it needs. Often, I advise people to read the same page of a book over and over again, and then to try and see what they can remember. Very often, people who lose concentration need to re-educate the mind and there is nothing more effective for this than meditating on one particular subject. My old teacher, Dr Leonard Allan, once taught us a little exercise that is useful when one is fed up and cannot concentrate sufficiently to learn. I, in turn, taught it to this particular gentleman and it helped him tremendously. Dr Allan told us that it was beneficial to try this universal law of spiritual levitation in order to help the concentration return. In so doing, we would also find out how enormous the power of God really is. When we practised the exercise, we sensed a stream of stronger energy entering our bodies and felt much better. It is therefore beneficial for people who have come to the stage of giving up praying, praying and praying again, and meditating, meditating and meditating again. This simple exercise is just one way of getting the concentration back to its original level.

Lie or sit in a comfortable position and place the right hand on top of the forehead and the left hand on the occiput (the little bone which sticks out right beneath the posterior region of the skull). Completely relax, breathing into the stomach and out through the mouth.

After carrying out this simple exercise, the gentleman wrote me a letter containing this little phrase, 'The love you liberate in your work is the only love you keep,' and said that my help had been remarkable. He felt I had been so caring, helpful and positive, that he could not help but feel positive too. For him and for others, this exercise has been of tremendous benefit.

A lady came to see me who was distressed and angry with God. She told me that her soul had almost been destroyed as she had prayed so hard to have a baby, without success. I helped both her and her husband understand their problem and work positively, after a little complication was taken taken care of. I was very touched by a letter she wrote me later, as she said that although she had not seen me for some time, she felt that her miraculous pregnancy was due to the help and remedies I had given her. She now had a lovely baby whose name meant 'calm and intelligent' and who very rarely cried. She felt this baby was a gift from God. The severe problems she was troubled with had cleared up and the new life created with this wonderful little baby taught them the value of life although, as she said, she had endured great upset. Her soul had been troubled by the fact that although doctors had told her there were no medical reasons why she could not conceive, nothing happened. God will work with us, not for us, and only in His time, and in matters of life and death one cannot force His hand. The most positive thing one can do is fully accept what happens to us in life and, from a medical point of view, do everything we possibly can to help. We need to learn to accept what life brings us and cope with life's ups and downs.

A little while ago, I lectured in front of about 500–600 people. During this lecture, I noticed a very well-dressed, elderly lady in her 90s, sitting in the front row. I looked at her and thought she was a typical example of a great soul, a soul that had been nourished and had learned in life, and even although her life had been very hard and she had no worldly possessions, she was very rich within herself. She had sacrificed her whole life to help the poor and needy in African countries, bringing those people hope for the future. In sacrificing herself this way she also enriched herself and enjoys very good health and a sound mind. She keeps herself up to date with everything going on around her and knows what it means to reflect the image of the God she serves, and has characteristics that would make one envious. Such a person encourages us to feel that life is worthwhile, that we should do what we can for others.

A fairly young lady came to consult me who was very spoiled. Her life revolved around herself and although she had never had to cope with any difficult situations during her life, she nevertheless had many emotional problems. She handed me an endless list she had prepared of ailments that were troubling her. This detailed her emotional problems of fear, panic, feeling unsafe, feeling trapped, unbalanced and irrational. It seemed that she suffered from panic attacks, agoraphobia, social phobia and depression, and had problems in her marriage which affected her family life and work. She also avoided trains, buses, cars, restaurants, the cinema, dentist, hairdresser and hospitals. Then she detailed her physical symptoms, which included hypersensitivity, sweating, tachycardia, tunnel vision, shaking, diarrhoea, confusion, nausea, breathlessness and feeling faint. She was unable to sit still, had no confidence in herself and said she had strong emotions in the stomach area. For such a relatively young woman, this was very sad. However, I had to start somewhere and as I felt that her body had become very toxic, I treated her with strong antioxidants and proceeded to cleanse her blood. Blood is a life elixir and it is extremely important nowadays to detoxify. Using the limited specialised equipment we have, it is surprising to see just how much waste material there is in blood. After that, I carried out some cranial osteopathy and bone symmetry, and prescribed beneficial remedies such as *avena sativa* and *zincum valerianicum*. She also needed considerable liver cleansing, which was helped with *Milk Thistle Complex* and complex vitamins, minerals and trace elements combined in *Optivite*, and I balanced her hormonal system with a great remedy called *Femcycle*. It was almost miraculous to witness the difference in this girl's life after only two weeks. Once more, this illustrates how much one can do when problems develop in the body and mind.

Another very emotional lady came to see me the other day and said she had achieved nothing in her life. She felt life was so hard and difficult that she could not carry on. When I talked to her, I felt she had suicidal tendencies, so I immediately gave her some *Emergency Essence* to calm her down, and then spoke to her. I said that although she felt very sorry for what she had not achieved in life, she had to keep going. I emphasised that a lot of overweight people have many problems – I gave Winston Churchill as an example, who after a life of setbacks, became prime minister at the age of 62. Then there was Henry Ford, who was made bankrupt about five times; Bill Gates, the founder of Microsoft, who was a college dropout and is now one of the richest people in the world; and Walt Disney who apparently had no vision but nevertheless formed Disneyland. There is a whole list of people who have fought very hard to achieve great things in life. I told her that from that moment on, she must decide to go forward and try, try and try again. One needs to have a goal and a vision in view before the answer will come.

This reminds me so much of my own father, who said that when he was imprisoned by the Germans it was not the physically strong people who coped with the torture, the concentration camps or the deportation, but the mentally and especially spiritually strong people who overcame such traumas, as he did himself. The more we feed ourselves spiritually and the stronger we become, the more problems we can face up to.

A simple little illustration which I dearly love comes to my mind. A very good friend and someone I respect highly, who went through deep emotional experiences during his life, said he always thought back to his first job, when he wanted to become a gardener. He was told to grow some little seedlings in six trays, which he did. Placed in the sunlight, the plants became strong, and flourished until something strange happened. His boss told him to move the plants into the dark cellar and allow them to wane. He looked in puzzlement at the boss and did not know why he wanted this done, but obediently did as he was instructed. He put the plants into the cellar, where slowly they deteriorated and withered, and eventually told his boss they were dying. When the plants were almost dead, his boss told him to bring them back out of the cellar, return them to the greenhouse where they could get plenty of sunlight and watch them carefully. He told him to make every effort to make the plants strong, and to inspect them further in a few weeks' time. At this point, he asked what was the purpose of the exercise he had just carried out. It was to make the plants strong: after the experience of nearly dying, they would fight for existence, grow to be their best and become very strong. That little message is a powerful one and a great lesson to us all, as it tells us that whatever happens in life and however sad our experiences might be, if they strengthen us we will become a better person in God's wonderful creation and will then be able to fulfil our purpose in life.

I recently visited an ex-policeman in prison. He asked me to come and see him as he was very distressed. He had never been a believer before but during his time in prison, he started to think about the meaning of life and became quite religious. He had read an expression which he very much agreed with: his soul was sore distressed. Previously he had turned against religion, as his wife was very religious and he didn't get on with her at all. Unfortunately, he came home one day, lost complete control when something didn't go his way and shot her dead in the presence of his son. Naturally, he was imprisoned and will spend many years in jail. I quoted him one of my favourite pieces from the bible: 'When a strong man armed keepeth his palace [meaning his heart], his goods are in peace' (St Luke, chapter 11, verse 21). When our hearts and souls become disconnected and weak, problems arise in our lives which can cause us to do the most dreadful things, as this man unfortunately discovered. I started to dig a bit into his medical history and found that there was, in fact, mental weakness in his family, and although he climbed to a fairly high rank in the police force, this caused him to carry out the tragic deed. I had a long chat with him and he understood what I was saying – that only by exercising our soul correctly can one make oneself strong and face daily life in a balanced way, so that instead of being depressed or miserable, one can deal with the most difficult battles.

On a lighter note, I am reminded of a gentleman who is probably one of the most wonderful people I have ever met in my life. He was elderly, with a white beard, had no earthly possessions, yet was the happiest man in the world. He was extremely intelligent and, at a particular point in his life, decided to devote his time to trying to help people so that they could be as happy as he was. He travelled all over the world and was a blessing to many. He was in close contact with nature and his Creator. I have never met anyone who was so happy and content with life, and who helped so many others lead a better life. One of the nicest memories I have is of a time he was walking up a hill with some colleagues, when some other people who saw him said to each other, 'He is talking to himself.' At this point, one of his colleagues said, 'Oh no, he doesn't talk to himself, he talks to God.' This man, who meditated and prayed so much, is a living example of how wonderful life can be when you have a view into the future, where everything will become new.

There are so many things that we can do to help ourselves when we are in turmoil. We have a rich treasury of herbs, plants, trees and roots that can help whenever necessary. One young missionary was very keen to go abroad into a missionary field. She spoke to her superiors, who arranged for her to go to a special place abroad. Initially, however, she was not keen to go there. She was a little troublesome but was sent nevertheless. Unfortunately, while out there she encountered problems with her colleagues, as she wasn't really willing to fit in. She had a disagreement with one of them and when she went to speak to a superior about it, she fell out with her too. Life became very difficult for everyone because of this young lady, who did not practise what she preached, which was to spread love that was beyond words. As she managed to upset so many people there, she was eventually told to leave and go home. Her heart was in the right place and she was not prepared to conform. When she returned home, she made a lot of fuss about what had taken place and was advised by her parents to write to the people she had upset and ask them for forgiveness. However, instead of following this advice, she wrote to them about how awful things had been for her while she was there. Her colleagues wrote back and said they would forgive her for what she had done, but she bluntly refused to ask for forgiveness. She went around telling everyone how awful it had been and that nobody cared about her or her rights, and things went from bad to worse. So she consulted me. I heard the whole story and she asked if there was anything I could do. I knew that I could probably speak to an uncle of one of my sons-in-law, who was in a high position, and that he might be able to intervene so that things could return to normal. When I wrote to ask if he would be prepared to do this, he said he would make enquiries into the matter. I then asked my patient to write to him, giving him all the facts, so that he could look into it. Some time later, when he had carried out investigations, he wrote back and said that unfortunately she had closed the door herself. He was very sorry, but he felt there was very little he could do until things were forgiven, but that forgiveness meant if one could forgive, one should forget. She still did not understand this message and was very bitter in herself, blaming all those who had been, as she said, 'so nasty to her'.

I was sorry for this girl as I felt that she had qualities that she could make use of, but life is also a question of sharing and loving others as one loves oneself. This is often where the struggle begins. I had a long talk with her, because I felt so much could be done to help. Luckily, the gardener had put some fresh St John's wort in my room that day. He knows that I love St John's wort with its flowers and leaves and I told her that perhaps we could learn a little lesson from one of the plant's namesakes, the apostle of love, St John. The ancient people must have known the benefits of St John's wort. It is the most loving plant. It almost shouts out to you, 'Please use me, I love you.' Breaking a leaf away from the stem of this flower, I said to her to look at the message the little leaf was trying to convey. It was virtually telling her to 'relax, let go and be at ease – all is forgiven because I love you'. The signature and characteristics of the plant are an indication that it works and this has been proven in my many years of working with it.

The most striking characteristic of the plant is obvious when you hold the leaf against the light. You will notice that miniscule pieces of light have become entrapped. When things need to be enlightened, especially in a situation like that of the young missionary, it tells us to be relaxed in every muscle and nerve, and enlighten the burdened mind. It is with that in mind that I prescribed this plant. This was a lesson for the young lady. She started to lighten up when I told her about it and, in addition to giving her St John's wort, I also prescribed a few other remedies. I later learned that, at her own expense, she returned to her colleagues to make a new start and has been happy ever since.

As I travel around and deal with many people, I often ask myself the question, 'What is the meaning of life?' Sometimes I feel there is much superficial understanding about mind, body and soul. In this often selfish world, where everybody wants to be more wealthy than the next person, it is good to examine one's life and realise that if we can live quite comfortably, we should accept that and try to be as happy as we can with what we have. In cases of chronic illness or emotional trauma, it is important to look at the methods that can be used to heal or open the door to a recovery, especially where our past lives have influenced our future.

We need to try and establish what is affecting our lives and why some people feel life is not worth living. It is no good hiding in a little corner where we feel safe and secure; we have to try and find answers as to why we are deeply unhappy or traumatised by a situation.

I received a letter from a lady I have known for many years. She said she found it very difficult to express her thoughts to me in writing, but felt she needed my help. She had experienced great unhappiness due to a dreadful situation she had endured at the hands of her husband, and had lived in a little comfort zone, with her life going from one crisis to another. Things continued along this road for over 20 years. She told me in the letter that although she had lived with this man for many years and he was often kind enough, he sometimes got so out of control that she felt he was going to kill her. It is awful when we see and hear of these unbelievable situations, but they do happen. She told me that he often tried to strangle her, but she had managed to survive. She now felt things had gone too far and one night, as he chased her with a can of hair spray in his hand threatening her, she begged him to end the violence. One evening when he arrived home late after having been drinking, he dragged her outside, forced her to lie down on a very rough part of the garden and proceeded to rape her. Not surprisingly this was extremely painful. He then further sexually abused her by indulging in the most obscene practices. She finally realised she could not cope any longer and left. She had reached the stage where she felt she could never go back to him, but her nervous system had gone completely to pieces and so she asked me for help. This had been such a traumatic time for her and there are certain diseases which can be triggered by trauma of the kind this poor woman had suffered. It had maimed her and affected her mobility. I had to use all kinds of treatments to settle her, like *Enhanced Nerve Factor*, acupuncture, some gentle cranial osteopathy and *Knot Grass Formula* from Bioforce, which luckily helped her joints tremendously. The continual stress over the years had brought this poor woman into a state of suffering as a result of the torture she had lived through, to the extent that she had lost all sense of reality. She deserved some happiness but others cannot create this for us, we have to work at it for ourselves and, therefore, she had to take steps towards building a new future.

Relaxation and meditation were important for her and when she discovered the true meaning of life, she found a combination of peace, power and inner calmness, and returned to her old self. I taught her my breathing exercise techniques, which were very beneficial, and told her to appreciate nature, of which she was a part. In addition, I asked her to imagine the ocean of life, where we are but a drop. If that drop is taken out of the ocean, it will soon dry up, and we will lose our sense of living. Emotions, whether positive or negative, carry a tremendously powerful energy. The more we control emotions with sensible thinking, the more we will come to understand our real inner feelings.

I remember a young girl who came to see me, whose life was ruled by her emotions. Since she was a young child, she had suffered from a very strange headache condition. She told me that, at the age of 23, in addition to taking dozens of aspirins, she also felt rejected by her family who were not sympathetic to the fact that she was always ill, because she had had all the tests and scans carried out and the results of these were negative. She had almost become addicted to aspirin. I told her the old story, which I have related in so many lectures, that if the church is on fire and the bells are ringing, you can stop the ringing but if you don't get the water hose out the fire will go on. I told her that she did the same with her headache: she took aspirins (she stopped the bells ringing), but she did not look at the underlying cause of her problem. She begged me to help her and I went over all the problems she had. When I carried out some cranial osteopathy, I felt there were tremendous tensions present. I then carried out very simple adjustments. The tension, which went from the spine right to the neck and to her head, was enormous – I have never felt so much tightness in all the 45 years I have been in practice. I said to her 'relax, relax and relax'. With some help, over time, she became well again. I discussed her problems with her, and the rejection that she felt so strongly about. Gradually, she changed from an extremely miserable girl to a very attractive person who is now very happily married.

It is a relief to let go of the emotional past and look at the reasons that tensions build up due to misunderstanding and thinking that we are worthless. I taught the girl a little piece of poetry by our national poet in Holland, P.A. de Genestet, which she found of great comfort. It tells us that when we look up to the sky and see the wonderful work of Creation – the moon and the stars which, with their silver glow, look at us – we are part of this. That piece of poetry ends with the wonderful words that our Creator gives all this to us in trust, we are all a part of it and he greets us all as his child. She really got great help from this poetry which, in Dutch, is very nicely worded. It made her feel a worthwhile person, a great part of the universe.

## MEDITATION
Practising visualisation exercises can bring immense benefit. Seeing ourselves as a new being and visualising what we would really like to be, evolving a higher sense to guide us through the awful situations that we can find ourselves involved in, will give a positive result. It is often a good idea to simply sit down and listen to our own inner voice, which wants to tell us so much and will guide us in many different situations.

Meditation is a form of relaxation. To meditate upon the positive aspect of a problem is a great help. One could say that prayer is possibly the most powerful form of meditation. Positive meditation and wanting to get well and to have the body in complete harmony is the best way to help the endocrine system, as it is not only physically and emotionally, but spiritually, of the greatest importance that balance is restored. The pituitary gland, which is so strongly linked with the cosmos, will react well to prayer and meditation. I see this often with patients who are under a lot of stress and anxiety.

A good form of meditation is as follows:

## First Part

Sit down in an easy chair, with your head resting and your feet flat on the floor. Breath calmly and hear your breath going in and out.

Now take a very deep breath in and, when expiring, say to yourself, 'Relax.'

Do this three times.

Now you are going to relax all the muscles of your body. Begin with your eyes and mouth. Squeeze your face tightly together and then suddenly let go. Feel a wave of relaxation travel down your body. Consciously relax your neck, shoulders, arms, hands, tummy, back, upper legs, the calves of your legs and feet.

When you have done this, try to think of a nice spot where you like to be – a lake, a mountainous area or a holiday spot, perhaps. Imagine you are there and stay with that memory for a couple of minutes.

This is the preparation for the exercise.

## Second Part

Now you are going to *see* your illness or problem. For illustration, I shall refer to the spine, but you should visualise whichever part of the body causes you problems, or whatever area in your life needs help. You are going to *see* with your mind's eye gloomy, grey patches in your spinal cord that do not look bright. You are going to *see* with your mind's eye how the bodily defences deal with it. You *see* blood vessels opening, bringing a flood of healthy blood loaded with vitamins. You *see* cells building, restoring the fatty layer around the nerve track. If you want to imagine the nerves as electric wires being restored with new insulation being put around them, then that is all right, as long as you *see* with your mind's eye how, with the help of vitamins, minerals and the body's own defence system, the spinal cord is restored to its original function.

Now, when you have finished this mental picture (and you may use your own imagination to suit the problem) you should see your illness as *weak* and your bodily defence as *strong*. You are going to see yourself quite strong again. You see yourself walking normally, full of vitality. Pat yourself on the back for having done so well. Breath deeply three times, then open your eyes.

Do this exercise three times a day: when you wake up, at lunchtime and before you go to sleep. Be in a quiet room. Never skip an exercise. Do not *force* yourself, just *see* it with your mind's eye. That is enough. What you're really doing is putting a new (and healthy) program into the computer. It may take you six to twelve months before the new program starts to work out in your body.

When we were children and had done something wrong, my mother used to say, 'Did you not listen to the little voice within you that told you not to do that?' Sometimes I wonder if we have lost the art of listening. In this extremely stressful world, where everyone is in such a hurry, do we still make time to listen? Although we often just drift through life, it is important to take time to listen to ourselves.

I will never forget when I was once asked to give my opinion on an elderly gentleman, to whom thousands of people flocked. As part of a team, we made enquiries about this gentleman and came to the conclusion that his success was purely due to the fact that he was an excellent listener. Without interruption, he let his patients talk and then offered them the right advice at the right time. That is a wonderful art, but the passion that he felt for his patients in advising them was such that he became very well known, which was evident from his long waiting lists.

Life is really very short. It is therefore important that we focus our attention on our ideals and make changes for the better, wherever possible. We have to spend time working on ourselves, living every day to the full, with the knowledge that we have been of help to others and shared some love in this often poor and selfish world. Sometimes that might be difficult but when we make a start, it is quite surprising how much we can achieve.

Once, while I was working in Hollywood, a very famous film star consulted me. I had a long conversation with her and she certainly understood the art of communication! She had an enormous energy outflow and I asked her what made her become so famous. She said it was determination. She continued, saying that when she started acting, she was quite unknown for some time, but she worked on it as she was determined to get to where she was now. She also carried out visualisation techniques and had a very positive attitude. She learned that she eventually became much more automatic in everything she was doing, with an energy and enthusiasm and a positive outlook in life, and also wanted to make other people happy. It was a wonderful conversation, which again emphasised the point that if one is determined, one can progress far in life.

Communication is important for the soul and, in order to

communicate properly, one has to put a great deal of personal feelings and emotion into it. It is wonderful to become our real selves, free from any negative influences from the world around us. Inner growth means looking into our soul and expressing the spirituality of who we really are and what we want to do with our relationships, our emotions and our life in general. The key is to become more aware in our own consciousness of what we are capable of achieving.

The other day I was consulted by a lovely young girl, whom I had known since she was a baby. I knew her parents had tremendous problems relating to alcohol and she said to me that because of the things she had encountered on the road that life had taken her, she too had turned to alcohol. She asked me if I felt the problem could be inherited. I enquired why she drank and she said that it was not the alcohol – she didn't really like it – but because she would suddenly find that she couldn't even sign her name because she felt so nervous and sometimes came out in a cold sweat. When her father admitted that he had started to drink for the same reason, she got a shock. She said it was probably that shock that helped her reduce her drinking, because it threw new light on the situation. She felt she had been given a reason as to the probable cause of her problems or inhibitions. So she came to me in order to help her overcome these problems, now that she realised why she had turned to alcohol. It is always a wonderful thing when one realises the cause of a problem, as very often the key to recovery is in one's own hands. I think that the knowledge of what had happened to her parents gave this girl an insight of how to help herself. Luckily, she recovered fully.

In our minds, we often have many questions we want answered. If we do not find an answer, we probably compensate by doing things that we should not, which might cause health problems. As a rule, the subconscious mind is very sensitive. It is also very receptive to suggestion and therefore even memory vibrations, however small they be, can be helped tremendously by a positive attitude. I do feel that, on this subject, it is important that even the smallest sensitivities are taken care of. Many people make light of this, but when I look at the many cases of allergy problems that can cause emotional distress to people, by using even the smallest homoeopathic remedy, a desensitisation can take place and the allergy can be cured. That is how quickly one can adjust certain problems. We must not forget that when one tiny electron vibrates, the whole universe is shaken. Even with little sensitivities, it is often the case that the smallest potency of a homoeopathic remedy can make the biggest difference.

There are a lot of people who, in their subconscious mind, have a fear of life caused by insecurity. Physical illness is often helped by a positive, realistic approach and yet, when people feel very insecure, with this fear and anxiety nestled in their subconscious mind, deep melancholy can develop. Often the fear will not disappear because the subconscious has erased the memory and it will be very difficult to convince the person with constant fear that everything is fine until balance or harmony can be found.

In such cases, I often have to use acupuncture to help alleviate the 'fear of fear', which becomes ingrained in the subconscious mind. There is very little that a practitioner can do, because the subconscious mind is subject to the relationship we have with our Creator, and is directed by the Creator. Faith is the key to overcoming problems which have become surrounded by fears and anxieties. Prayer, meditation and coming into contact with nature is the best possible help.

A very well-known writer once said,

> How ever far into the boundless realms of the unconscious we may succeed in carrying the victorious invasion of the intellect, I fancy that we shall always reach a point eventually at which the only practical policy consists of taking the unconscious on its own terms, allowing the unconscious to speak for itself. It depends on our conscious mind what kind of actions we make and what motives to control.

I once experienced this with a very high-powered banker, who was always surrounded by fear because of his dealings with vast sums of money. When he came to me with these huge problems, I told him it was healthy for him to want to do his best – and that is as much as anyone can do – but that he must learn to accept matters. Often the problem then solves itself. It makes no difference to the outcome if you lie day and night worrying about something that is temporary. It is much more important to invest in our future, in our health and well-being, because if we don't do that the other area will fail anyway.

We often see with people who have become hypochondriacs, or suffer from any kind of neurosis, that they have lost all sense of reality in life and need to be properly directed in a way that lets them rediscover themselves. It is important to rid them of the strain within, which can sometimes drive them to destruction. I believe very strongly that an understanding of the powers that exist in every one of us can heal, as long as these powers are intelligently directed towards a positive action.

Healing is in oneself, and there is a wonderful passage in one of the oldest books of the Bible, Ecclesiastes (which is well worth reading). It says that healing, not only for the soul but also for the mind and body, becomes necessary. I have often seen that miracles really do happen. I once looked at a young girl who was not only physically ill, but was mentally very distressed. I asked her to read my book, *Body Energy*. I told her simply to do for herself the healing I explain there, and a miracle happened. She came back to me and said she did it faithfully, and admitted that she made a speedy recovery when she started to believe that it would work. Such positive thoughts, believing that things work, are essential with either orthodox or alternative medicine. Divine love only wants to help us heal and restore, so that we can enjoy the great miracle of life.

I love that little quotation from the Bible for people who are always scared, very often for themselves, and have a great fear of the future. This has often helped others as well as myself: 'There is no fear in love; perfect love casteth out fear.' When fears are removed and trust takes their place, disease will leave us. We just have to trust and not only have faith in our Creation but also in ourselves. That will often bring about the healing that is necessary for the vast majority of people who think very negatively. So many people persist in looking on the black side of things and, as a result of that, one loses security and becomes apathetic. It is absolutely essential to replace negative thoughts with positive ones.

A girl who was quite a famous ballet dancer consulted me a few days ago. She came from a very loving family (I knew her parents), and when she became famous, she was asked to dance in Paris. While there, and without the knowledge of her parents, she grew homesick – she missed the love that had surrounded her at home and made her who she is. Slowly, her health deteriorated, she became lonely and anorexic. By the time her parents found out, her weight had plummeted to around six stone. They brought her to see me. I spoke to her and it soon became apparent that it was the love from home that she was missing, and although she had a glorious and rewarding life in Paris, there was no love, which no amount of success could replace. I had to work a lot on her as she was severely anorexic, but with the help of *avena sativa*, oats extract, zinc and extra vitamins, she recovered. But it was the love of her family that really returned her to her former self. This made me realise once again that it is very often love that keeps us ticking over. I was brought up with a lot of love, especially from my mother, and every time that I feel down, I try to imagine that she is looking around the door to encourage me and show me that her love, which I experienced so much while she was alive, is still present, because the connection is still there to offer me encouragement.

Happiness is based on great love, and it is obvious that healthy people are a lot happier than unhealthy people. It is quite evident that when one feels well, one can show the tremendous love that is given to every one of us as long as we develop it. It is a good idea to exercise one's health with a little bit of self-awareness, realising that we are individuals and should not compare ourselves to others. As long as the example is positive and we redevelop in our conscious mind an idea of what is necessary to become a better person, we can be sure that the subconscious mind, which is directed by God, will show us the right road to take.

When we become more aware of ourselves, we become more aware of the needs of others, and that teaches us compassion. It is a particular quality that people who have learned to love and be kind possess. It is often when life becomes a reality that we rediscover how much is in store for all of us.

It is said so beautifully, 'Be still, and know that I am God,' and in the stillness and quietness, we will discover that God wants to be in our hearts. That is really food for the soul and will bring the spirituality we often need so much. To repeat, although we are but a drop in the ocean, we still belong to that ocean, and to this great universe which William Blake described so well in his poetry:

> To see a World in a Grain of Sand
> And a Heaven in a Wild Flower
> Hold Infinity in the Palm of your Hand
> And Eternity in an Hour.

The conscious awareness that all this is entrusted to us makes us thankful for the great gift of life that is given to us at birth and that we want to enjoy, in body, mind and soul, as much as we can.

I am now coming to the end of the book. At the beginning of this final part, my very good friend asked me how she could become more spiritual and help others. God has given us the gift of life and the capacity to show love. The key to love is to become unselfish, more compassionate, more merciful, more forgiving and, filled with this spiritual understanding, to realise that love is not only given to oneself, but embraces the whole of the human race. When love fulfils all, it is perfect and in harmony with Creation. Love is the name of God, for God is love and love is eternal, and will heal so many troubles.

Life cannot always be filled with sunshine and sometimes there will be shadows. We cannot always be happy. Carl Jung wrote,

> Even a happy life cannot be without a measure of darkness and the word happiness would lose its meaning if it were not balanced by sadness. All these experiences are necessary to form us as a person, to give us more personality and character that shows how we stood the test in shaping up to life.

The heart is measured by love. Do you have a loving heart? This love should be not only for our husband, wife, partner or children, but for all around us. Love will overcome anger, jealousy and hatred, and all negative thoughts, by a positive decision made by the heart. Even a wounded heart can be restored by love. Our soul is filled with it and, indeed, love will help us become more spiritual, as my friend so dearly wished. God's abundance has no limits. We can drink from this tremendous source of love, light and joy, and come to understand what perfect peace means.

God created the most important thing on the first day: the spiritual light that surrounds every one of us. We have to learn to walk in that light, and Christ gives the perfect example, exhibiting a love for God, each other and nature. If we can do this, one day all will be new.

# INDEX